T0327818

Chinese Medicine for the Mind

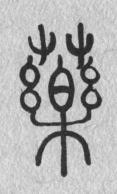

Chinese Medicine for the Mind

A Science-Backed Guide to Improving Mental Health with Traditional Chinese Medicine

Nina Cheng
and Contributors

FAIR WINDS

Quarto.com
© 2024 Quarto Publishing Group USA Inc.
Text © 2024 Nina Cheng

First Published in 2024 by Fair Winds Press, an imprint of The Quarto Group,
100 Cummings Center, Suite 265-D, Beverly, MA 01915, USA.
T (978) 282-9590 F (978) 283-2742

Fair Winds Press titles are also available at discount for retail, wholesale, promotional, and bulk purchase. For details, contact the Special Sales Manager by email at specialsales@quarto.com or by mail at The Quarto Group, Attn: Special Sales Manager, 100 Cummings Center, Suite 265-D, Beverly, MA 01915, USA.

28 27 26 25 24   1 2 3 4 5

ISBN: 978-0-7603-9125-9

Digital edition published in 2024

eISBN: 978-0-7603-9126-6

Library of Congress Control Number (LCCN) available.

Design and Page Layout: Studio Chenchen | studiochenchen.com
Cover Image: Studio Chenchen | studiochenchen.com
Illustration: Yi-Wen Hsu | Studio Chenchen

Printed in China

The information in this book is for educational purposes only. It is not intended to replace the advice of a physician or medical practitioner. Please see your health-care provider before beginning any new health program. The effectiveness of the remedies presented is not guaranteed.

ACKNOWLEDGMENTS

This book is the culmination of the work of a number of scholars and practitioners, including those recognized for their incomparable expertise in the history and practice of Chinese medical psychology. I would especially like to thank Brandt Stickley, LAc, for lending his decades of expertise treating mental health conditions to this book.

LEAD CONTRIBUTOR

Brandt Stickley, LAc

OTHER CONTRIBUTORS

Alexus McLeod, PhD
Shanshan Gao, Master of Clinical Medicine, PhD
Daniel Spigelman, Bachelor of Medicine (China)

SPECIAL THANKS TO

Dolly Yang, PhD
Josh Paynter, LAc
Z'ev Rosenberg, LAc

CON

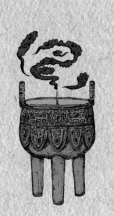

TENTS

INTRODUCTION

The best-selling herbal formula in all of Chinese medicine—some estimate that it comprises 45 percent of all herbal formula sales—is for mood disorders, including depression and anxiety. First recorded in a pharmacopeia compiled by the Imperial Medical Bureau during the Northern Song dynasty (960–1127 CE), it is an herbal medicine that has been popular for over a thousand years, meticulously recorded in case studies by Chinese medicine physicians over the centuries. This formula rose to prominence during an era of ancient China that represented the ultimate in modernization, sophistication, and urbanization, with a gross domestic product three times larger than that of Europe. Marco Polo, a merchant from Europe's most sophisticated city, Venice, visited China at the tail end of the Song dynasty and was overwhelmed with its splendor and technology, calling one of its cities "beyond dispute, the finest in the world." To cope with the stresses and anxieties of such an increasingly cosmopolitan and mentally demanding lifestyle, especially as a new class of candidates took up preparations for the hypercompetitive Imperial Exam, those overwhelmed by modern stressors often turned to herbal medicine. This formula provides some insight into how herbal prescriptions were developed in ancient China, and how timeless many of our struggles are.

In more recent times, this formula has shown excellent efficacy through extensive clinical research using randomized, double-blind, controlled trials, including one that showed it outperformed prescription selective serotonin reuptake inhibitor (SSRI) medications in reducing anxiety with depression. It is also extremely safe, with no known side effects found after a systemic review of multiple trials. It is widely available today, in powder, pill, tablet, granule, and raw herb form, with most bottles starting at around $10. Despite these facts, this treatment has not attracted widespread attention and is completely unknown to most of the West.

This example is only one of the many herbal formulas for mental health in traditional Chinese medicine that share a similar story: They are time-tested formulas with an excellent safety profile and known efficacy. However, there seems to be a pervasive misconception that Chinese medicine is not equipped to treat mental health conditions. In the United States, Chinese medicine is mostly known for treating musculoskeletal injuries, pain, and infertility, as well as chronic diseases that may not have solutions in Western medicine. Acupuncture, which has begun to be integrated into mainstream medicine, also overwhelmingly dominates Chinese medicine practice in the West, and extensive knowledge of herbal medicine is rare, even among licensed practitioners. Only a small percentage of Chinese medicine practitioners in the United States receive training in herbal medicine, an unfortunate situation considering that in China, herbal medicine is considered the more effective treatment modality.

This book's goal is to introduce practical and accessible solutions within Chinese medicine for mental health and shine a light on its incredible ability to understand and treat our mind-body imbalances. I discuss insomnia, depression, anxiety, attention deficit hyperactivity disorder (ADHD) and lack of focus, brain fog, and trauma using language that is easily understandable from a Western perspective, even without a full understanding of traditional Chinese medicine's terms and concepts. An historian's overview is also included for each condition, highlighting how each was understood and treated throughout ancient China, as well as patterns from a clinical approach and corresponding herbal medicine recommendations. More than just herbal medicine, however, this book also includes proven methods across multiple modalities, including food therapy, acupressure, music therapy, qigong, dao-yin, and even feng shui, accompanied by clinical studies when available.

Chinese Medicine for the Mind reflects the vision and methods of The Eastern Philosophy, an online Chinese medicine apothecary, in combining clinical studies with a historical source–based approach to understanding mental health from a Chinese medicine standpoint. I launched The Eastern Philosophy as a passion project on Instagram in late 2019, sharing my long-form science and history-based research on traditional Chinese medicine, as well as other time-honored wellness practices within Chinese culture that I grew up with. The Eastern Philosophy eventually turned into an online shop and is now one of the largest social media accounts about Asian medicine today. My mission is to build trust and educate those unfamiliar with this medical system in an authentic way that honors its history and culture, through high-quality content from experts. This book similarly takes an expert-led approach, and it is the culmination of the work of a number of scholars and practitioners, including those recognized for their incomparable expertise in Chinese medicine psychology.

While you may notice that Chinese medicine has surged in terms of consumer interest, many of those on the academic side are aware that there is currently a crisis in Chinese medicine: Multiple Chinese medicine institutions in the West have shuttered their doors in the past year due to rising costs and low enrollment, and many traditional medicine clinics and manufacturers have closed down, driven by a general lack of interest from the younger generations to take over. My hope is that books like this one will help introduce Chinese medicine to Western readers in an approachable way and demonstrate how this millennia-old medical system is more relevant and needed than ever. Thank you for helping keep this ancient tradition alive.

Why Traditional Chinese Medicine and Why Now?

Traditional Chinese medicine (TCM) is the oldest continuously used system of medicine that exists today. For more than five thousand years, Chinese practitioners have used herbal formulas and traditional healing modalities to treat countless human ailments. While herbal medicine is used in hundreds of cultures around the world, the practice in China is the most extensively documented and cataloged.

Although Chinese medicine has existed in the West for the past few decades, TCM has recently reached a major turning point. It has increasingly gained acceptance in global health care, bolstered by a surge of high-quality studies on the efficacy of TCM remedies as well as an endorsement from the World Health Organization (WHO); their influential International Statistical Classification of Diseases and Related Health Problems now includes TCM remedies. Furthermore, the 2015 Nobel Prize in Medicine was awarded to a Chinese scientist for her research based on a classical Chinese medicine cure for malaria from a fourth-century text. Before this, traditional medical knowledge (from any country) had never even been on the radar for Nobel Prize prospects, creating a seismic shift in international attention on TCM.

Chinese medicine relies on accumulated experience and inherited wisdom. Although folk medicine practitioners did and continue to exist, the core of Chinese medicine knowledge is passed down primarily from learned doctors, with thousands of ancient texts from these physicians documenting the most effective herbal formulas, treatment protocols, and patient case studies going back to the early Han dynasty, around 200 BCE. According to the historical records of one regional school of medicine, known as the Xin'an Medical School, starting from the Jin dynasty (266–420 CE), Xin'an physicians compiled about 800 medical books on a wide array of human health topics for virtually every bodily system and theory of practice, including 210 books on internal medicine, 24 books on gynecology, and 77 books on case studies.

Although part of the increasing popularity of traditional Chinese medicine is connected to a growing interest in wellness and leading a more holistic lifestyle, another part of its popularity is also due to a loss of faith in modern health care. With an alarming proportion of reversals and drug recalls, major gaps in Western biomedicine's ability to treat diseases that are chronic or psychological in nature, and increased awareness of financial incentives corrupting clinical data, there has been growing criticism of modern medicine. This "has prompted some skeptics to look beyond the confines of our own traditions" just as more academics have "begun to focus their research on China, where a wealth of written sources permits tracing a lively tradition of health care over several thousand years," according to the influential historian Paul Unschuld.

The notion of wellness has been a trend in the West for the past decade, but wellness has been an obsession in China since antiquity, and Chinese medicine originated from the ancient Daoist preoccupation with longevity and immortality. According to Chinese medicine author Giovanni Maciocia, "Due to the Daoist masters' research into herbal remedies, acupuncture, and breathing exercises to attain 'immortality,' or longevity, we now have a rich inheritance of herbal and acupuncture treatments as well as breathing exercises and life's 'hygiene' rules aimed at strengthening a weak constitution. The complex of such Daoist teachings is called Yang Sheng in Chinese, that is, 'nourishing life.'"

How to Use This Book

There are hundreds of books that go into depth explaining the fundamentals of traditional Chinese medicine, aimed at both practitioners and a general audience. This book does not focus as much on theory but rather more on applied practice, particularly related to mental health. I encourage you to start by reading the first three chapters, which discuss the basics of Chinese medicine treatments, including important information on herbal formulas. Then read the chapters that are relevant or interesting for your particular needs. Citations, organized by chapter, start on page 150.

I hope this book will serve as a useful handbook to help improve your mental health and general well-being as well as illuminate the culture, history, and science behind the Chinese medicine tradition.

Note:
None of the formulas presented here are meant to be prepared on your own. The formulas in this book are widely available in standardized prepared form, such as pills, granules, and tablets. It is not generally recommended to procure individual raw herbs for decocting for various reasons covered in chapter 3.

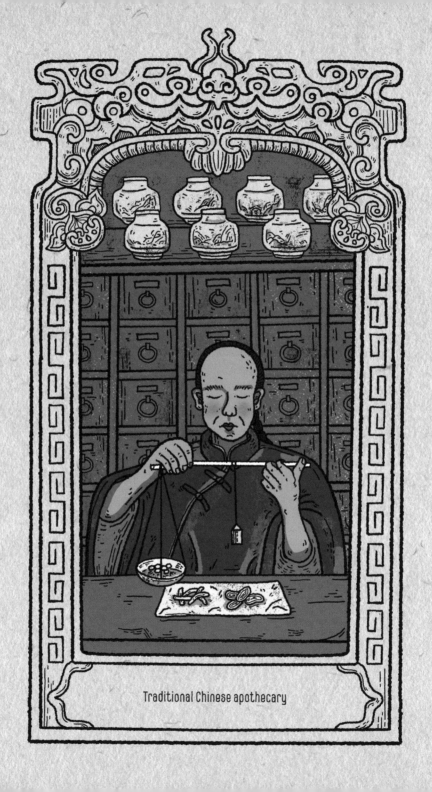

Traditional Chinese apothecary

CHAPTER 1

A HISTORICAL OVERVIEW OF TRADITIONAL CHINESE MEDICINE

Mental illnesses have been among the conditions discussed by the Chinese medical tradition since its beginnings in the early centuries BCE. In fact, the Chinese tradition preserves one of the oldest discussions of mental illness in medical literature across the world. It is likely the first tradition to recognize various mental health and behavioral disorders as illnesses with treatments that can be provided by physicians.

This chapter reviews the history of mental health in Chinese medicine, dispels some of the most common misconceptions about Chinese medicine, and considers how science and spirituality fit into this medical system today.

The earliest specifically medical account of mental illness found in the Chinese tradition is contained in the *Huangdi Neijing* 黃帝內經 (*Inner Classic of the Yellow Emperor*), compiled in the first century BCE and including material likely older than this. In the *Lingshu Jing* 靈樞經 (*Spiritual Pivot Classic*), one of two texts compiled in the *Huangdi Neijing* collection, there is a chapter specifically covering "madness" (kuang 狂) as an illness (bing 病), and describing its symptoms and treatments, with other passages in the text discussing its causes. "Madness" in the text can be associated with a cluster of illnesses with symptoms associated with conditions today referred to as anxiety, bipolar disorder, and depression (among others).

The *Lingshu Jing* describes madness as an illness that often begins with milder forms, such as sadness, forgetfulness, and fear, and that can progress to more severe conditions with manic symptoms, such as getting little sleep, not eating, considering oneself "high and valuable," and using insulting, harsh, or wild words. More severe conditions such as schizophrenia are also suggested by other descriptions of the symptoms of madness in the text, such as "having false visions," "hearing false sounds," and "seeing ghosts and spirits."

According to the early medical texts, the Heart or Heart-Mind (xin 心) and the spirit (shen 神) are the individual's components most affected by mental illness. The *Huangdi Neijing* attributes mental illnesses most directly to disorders concerning qi (氣), the vital energy (sometimes translated as "psychophysical substance") contained in and transferred through the five Organ systems of the human body—Heart, Lung, Spleen, Kidney, and Liver. (Note that these refer to a metaphorical part of a traditional Chinese medical visceral system, not the actual bodily organ.) When qi is depleted, blocked, or otherwise not moving correctly between the Organs, a variety of physical and mental illnesses emerge. Qi can be of a yin (陰) (still, yielding) or yang (陽) (active, powerful) quality. When insufficient quantity of a type of qi is present in a particular Organ, illness can result and can be caused by the environment, injury, and even our own activity.

In the case of mental illnesses, specifically, the *Huangdi Neijing* points to two main lifestyle causes: the overabundance of emotion, which can be situational or chronic, and improper activity generating excessive heat, such as a faulty diet or overwork, causing qi to be distributed improperly.

The *Huangdi Neijing*'s analysis of mental illness formed the core of the Chinese medical tradition's understanding of these illnesses and their causes through most of Chinese history, until the contemporary period. At the same time, new treatments have continually emerged through the development of the tradition. In the classic third-century CE text *Shanghanlun* 傷寒論 *(Treatise on Injuries from Cold and Miscellaneous Diseases)*, compiled by physician Zhang Zhongjing (150–219 CE) circa 200 CE, madness was understood to have often been caused by the generation of excessive or displaced heat, and the text offered a number of herbal medicines that could be helpful in treating mental illnesses of the kind associated with heat. For this reason, many remedies were prescribed to reduce heat.

We also find robust discussion of mental illness, particularly via the concept of "madness" (kuang) in early Chinese philosophical texts. There are a host of different positions on kuang, from the moralist position of Confucian texts, such as the *Xunzi* (third century BCE), which argue that such illnesses can result from failure to properly develop oneself morally, to the position found in the *Zhuangzi* (fourth through second century BCE), which celebrates madness (along with what we would now consider concepts of neurodivergence and disability) as representation of alternative perspectives on the world, allowing one to recognize the limited and provisional nature of any given worldview. These positions all influence the medicalized conception of kuang that emerges in the early Chinese medical tradition.

In the twelfth century, new concepts of madness began to emerge that focused on the Heart-Mind as their functional source, linked to disorders of qi in the chest (connected to the Lung in particular). In addition to kuang, medical texts of this period also include discussion of the mental illness dian (癲), which appears as something akin to depression or lethargy and is sometimes combined with kuang, and was often understood to involve seizures as well as mental and behavioral symptoms.

An interesting aspect of Chinese discussions of mental illness was the view—found in numerous texts throughout the history of the Chinese intellectual tradition more broadly—that features of one's environment and community could play contributing roles in bringing about illness as well as in treatment of illness. This was tied to a focus on preventive medicine, even from the earliest texts such as *Huangdi Neijing*. Prevention of mental illness is tied to organization and proper treatment of the body and mind, and engagement in activity with an aim toward maintaining harmony between the operation of the body's components, the other aspects of the individual, and the community.

According to the *Huangdi Neijing*, we can avoid mental illnesses caused by overabundant emotion by restraining the mind and avoiding conditions for the generation of certain dangerous emotions. The text teaches that you should, for example, "let the mind have no anger," with the idea that anger is volatile and can disrupt the mind in ways that lead to illness. The ideas developed in the Chinese medical tradition are found in a host of other texts as well, particularly those dealing with ethics, an important corollary of medicine in Chinese intellectual tradition. A passage from the ancient philosophical text *Guanzi* 管子 explains that both pleasure and anger have the potential to disorder the mind, leading it to "lose its original form."

The recognition in the Chinese medical tradition that there are ways we can use our bodies and minds that overtax or harm them and can lead to mental illness is an important insight of the tradition. The various treatment strategies found in the tradition for mental illness were developed over 2,500 years and include preventive strategies such as meditation and lifestyle changes, as well as medicinal interventions such as herbal recipes, emetics, and well-known physical techniques such as acupuncture and moxibustion, among a host of others. The Chinese medical tradition has the longest and most sustained tradition of discussion and treatment of mental illness in the world and has an enormous amount to contribute to such treatment today.

Science and Chinese Medicine

There is often a misconception that traditional Chinese medicine is unsubstantiated, mystical, unscientific, and illogical, even among those in the medical profession. Western doctors generally have no training or familiarity with traditional Chinese medicine, or any kind of herbal medicine, and often are completely unaware of any alternatives to the biomedical arsenal. Yet, thousands of all-natural TCM remedies exist, many of which have been shown in double-blind, placebo-controlled studies to be effective, some even outperforming synthetic drugs—and often without the side effects, addictive potential, or high cost of these pharmaceuticals.

The notion that there are clinical studies on Chinese medicine at all often shocks people, who seem to equate TCM with something between homeopathy and sorcery. There have, in fact, been placebo-controlled clinical studies on Chinese medicine since the 1960s, and studies in the West since the 1970s. It could now even be said that medical governing bodies in China are obsessed with clinical studies, sometimes to the dismay of practitioners.

While thousands of trials exist examining the efficacy of Chinese medicine treatments, including many individual herbal formulas, large-scale human trials—which are standard with pharmaceutical drugs—are less common in TCM. This is due, unfortunately, to the expense of large-scale human studies typically funded by pharmaceutical companies, which are incentivized to do so to bring a patented drug to market and profit from its sales. There will always be fewer studies available on herbal medicine, because herbs are not patentable drugs and so provide no incentive for companies to fund expensive, large-scale human trials. In contrast, any clinical trials on herbal medicine tend to be driven by pure scientific or medical interest, not profits.

I include a number of clinical studies to support the efficacy of Chinese herbal remedies and other healing modalities discussed throughout this book in an effort to assure readers that many Chinese medicine remedies have not only been time-tested for over 2,500 years but have also gone through more rigorous modern scientific testing over the last few decades.

Spirituality in Chinese Medicine

It should be noted that many aspects of traditional Chinese medicine as it is practiced today are incorrectly assumed by a Western audience to be "spiritual" (and, therefore, in opposition to science), when they are, in fact, simply using different language and nomenclature. Partially, this may be due to the challenges of translation and the difficulty of finding words in English that precisely define concepts from another culture. A frequently encountered example is the common

translation for the Chinese character "天." Pronounced "tian" and often found in texts on Chinese medicine. In Chinese, its meaning can be of the physical sky, the universe, or the entirety of nature. Sometimes, it has a religious implication as the place where deities live. Regardless, tian is almost always translated into English as "heaven," infusing every context with a divine implication that is not necessarily intended.

Other times, the metaphorical language of Chinese medicine, or the continuity of terminology that originated in ancient times, can give readers the impression that TCM remains heavily steeped in mysticism. As observed by Paul Unschuld, "A casual reading of the texts of the medicine of systematic correspondence reveals that here, too, diseases are occasionally caused by the 'malevolent'... in particular, the term hsieh 邪 (evil, harmful) that is used for all pathogenic agents. However, the meaning of the old term has been transformed. Evil itself is no longer embodied by demons, but rather by abstract as well as empirically visible influences and emanations."

You'll likely find references to "evil wind" or "pre-heaven energy" in most contemporary books about Chinese medicine. It's important to remember that these are not describing literal concepts.

While in the twentieth and twenty-first centuries Chinese medicine has increasingly moved away from its religious roots, there are certainly remnants of a spiritual, shamanistic tradition that still exist, although they are hard to find, especially in the West. According to a sixteenth-century text compiled by Xu Chunfu called *The Complete Compendium of Ancient and Contemporary Medical Work*,

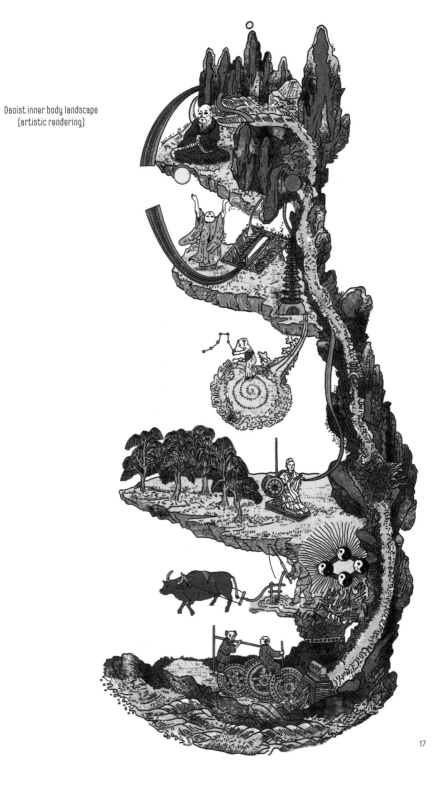

Daoist inner body landscape
(artistic rendering)

which profoundly elucidated medical theories, Xu explains the disadvantages of taking only medicine without utilizing spells during illness, or only seeking a shaman and not taking medicine:

> For the treatment of illnesses arising from the harmful effects of evil there are both spells, which eliminate all uncertainty [as to a possibly demonic origin of the affliction], and drugs, which require a careful investigation of depletions and surpluses, an examination of phlegm and fire [in the organism], as well as a consideration of the severity [of the individual case]. When both therapeutic approaches are combined, inner and outer [elements] are unified, and a rapid recovery from the illness is assured.
>
> He who consults only a shaman and utilizes no drugs of any kind shall not recover from his illness, for there is no underlying principle to bring about the cure. He who takes only drugs and does not consult a shaman to eliminate all uncertainty, shall be cured, but the recovery will be slow. Therefore both inner and outer elements must be treated simultaneously, as this will produce a rapid success.

Chinese shamanic and Daoist medicine are medical systems that may use incantations, talismans, and spells alongside herbs and acupuncture to heal afflictions.

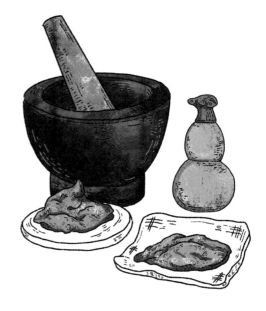

Daoist Medicine: Interview with Josh Paynter

Josh Paynter is a traditional Chinese medicine practitioner, twenty-second-generation Daoist priest, and co-abbot of Parting Clouds, a Daoist temple.

Q: I often hear of people in Asia seeking Daoist medicine practitioners when they suffer from certain conditions—especially mental health conditions—that haven't responded well to Western or TCM interventions. What approaches does Daoist medicine have to treat mental health conditions that are distinct from TCM?

A: The TCM and Daoist approaches to mental health are quite distinct. The mind, after all, is the primary concern of much of the Daoist cultivation tradition. We have robust systems for understanding the human mind and how the spectrum of mental health is far more diverse than "well" and "unwell." Daoist interactions with consciousnesses consider a host of potentials. The religious domain has the availability of the metaphysical, the metaphorical, the mundane, the celestial, the demonic, and so much more. These ontologies can overlap with those found in the framework of TCM approaches to psychology or mental health, but the methods employed in TCM are all ultimately reduced to those same methods employed in the physiological frameworks. In Daoist medicine (DM), the methods employed are specifically mind-focused or, more specifically, spirit-focused. Words, images, songs, deities, prayer, and ritual are the methodologies of Daoist medicine. Even if acupuncture and herbs are also simultaneously employed, the preeminent methods of the Daoist are rooted in prayer, spoken, written, or enacted in ritual form. It is in this domain of ritual and prayer that the main distinction between TCM and Daoist medicine lies.

Q: It seems DM practitioners predominantly focus on the use of incantations and talismans to treat patients. Are there any healing DM practices people can do on their own at home?

A: Daoist medicine requires a Daoist to perform it. This means that Daoist medicine is really only Daoist medicine if an ordained or otherwise initiated member of a Daoist medicine lineage is performing the healing method. This, however, is not an impasse. A great resource for the acquisition of cultural practices is the annual *Tongshu* or *Chinese Almanac*. There are usable talismans, daily proscriptions for things to avoid (bad luck), daily advice for things to do (good luck), divination methods, and so much more. As is the case with any medicine, as one's needs become more specific or severe, it is advisable to seek the care or interventions of those who are qualified to provide such.

Q: Feng shui seems to be one of the practices that DM practitioners may prescribe, distinct from TCM practitioners. Do you have feng shui recommendations to improve general mental health, or for people suffering from trauma?

A: Feng shui is definitely something we prescribe. Our method differs from the well-known applications that employ the manipulation or remediation of objects or architecture in physical space. Our method is a specialized branch of calculated feng shui that employs the calendar as the functional tool—we are concerned with the dimension of time more than of space. The moment that a patient notices a problem, the moment they contact us, the moment they employ the cure we prescribe, all of these moments in time are taken into consideration when we make our calculations. To intervene, we need to understand the causes, which requires a temporal map of the patient's life from birth until the appearance of the current condition. All of this can be pertinent when defining a course of treatment.

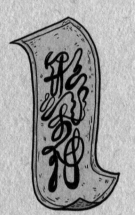

In a more general sense, we believe mental health and healing from trauma both require a setting that does not exacerbate any disturbances. Regardless of the size of one's domestic space, or its location or orientation or any other geomantic factor, there are some general approaches that can be a factor in improving mental health. The home should reflect the general aspirations of the patient. Images, words, colors, or objects that are cause for discomfort, alarm, uncomfortable memories, or other disturbances should be modified or removed. Being sensitive to things around us and making changes as needed are typical Daoist practices.

Q: There's been a trend in TCM to take on a more biomedical approach, classifying disorders with biomedical terms and substantiating treatments with clinical studies. What are we losing if we practice only a biomedical TCM, stripped of any spiritual component?

A: Human wellness cannot be fully realized without the attendance of all of our potentials. All physiological dimensions and systems, all cognitive and psychological aspects, all spiritual and metaphysical domains are essential to our completeness. Religion and spirituality are very hard to reconcile with medicine as it exists today. Modernity and industrial realities coupled with the urgencies of capitalism are the backdrop in the struggle to maintain spiritual dimensions within medicine in its current applications. TCM is not immune to these forces. Fortunately, TCM has the infrastructure to yet again receive and reintegrate the legacy of Chinese spiritual medicine. The Daoist community has carried forth and preserved these traditions and practices. It is my goal, and the goal of others in my community, to responsibly facilitate this reintegration.

Conclusion

From reading this chapter, you have now been introduced to the 2,500-year history of mental health in Chinese medicine. An important takeaway from the insights of ancient Chinese physicians and intellectuals is that mental and physical health can be harmed via our community or environment, as well as by the ways we overtax ourselves. You may have been surprised to learn that there are a vast number of clinical studies on Chinese medicine remedies, including thousands of double-blind, placebo-controlled trials since the 1960s, as well as how spirituality, which certainly played a part in the history of Chinese medicine, has largely been stripped from traditional Chinese medicine but still exists in shamanic or Daoist medicine.

In the next chapter, you will begin to learn about the most relevant aspects of Chinese medicine theory, including the Five Phases, and how the Organ systems fit in. For those new to Chinese medicine, the correspondence of Organs to emotions can be one of the most confusing and seemingly arbitrary aspects. But a firm grasp of these foundations will allow you to view Chinese medicine—and perhaps even the world around you—in a new light.

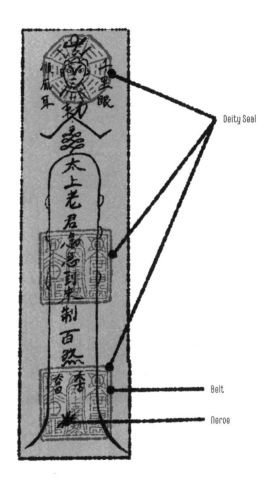

Daoist talisman (artistic rendering)

Deity Seal

Belt

Neroe

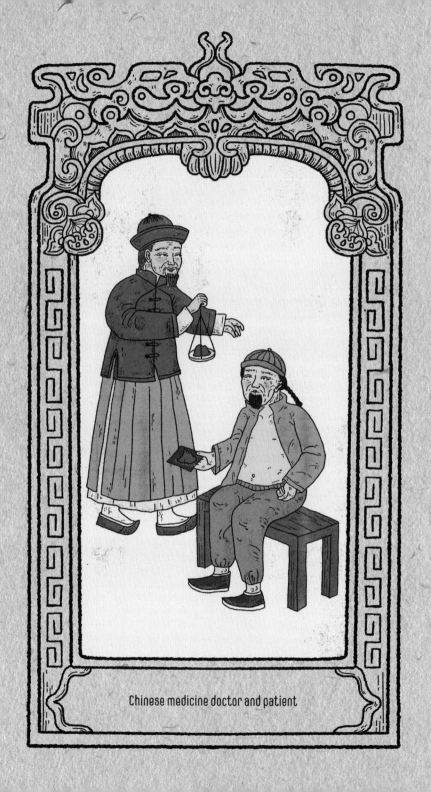

Chinese medicine doctor and patient

CHAPTER 2

EMOTIONS AND MENTAL HEALTH IN CHINESE MEDICINE

This chapter introduces the foundations of Chinese medicine theory as well as its unique approach to mental health. The TCM approach is extremely different from the Western medical approach to treating mental health, in which patients are given strictly psychiatric diagnoses that are perceived as stigmatized and chronic, and often presented only with pharmaceutical options for treatment that may be accompanied by major side effects. Instead, and unlike Western medicine, in TCM, conditions such as depression are recognized as one symptom in a broader diagnosis of imbalance, categorized by an indication that combines both physical and psychological symptoms: Liver Qi Stagnation, for example. Unlike the Western dualistic nature of "body and mind," Chinese medicine does not have these divisions. Historically, there has been no split between disorders of the mind and those of the body as there is in Western medicine. Chinese medicine physicians recognize that the mind and body are interconnected, and symptoms—as well as treatments—comprise all aspects of a person's experience.

For example, someone who suffers from anxiety may find that it subsequently causes intestinal distress (such as loose stools); a Chinese herbal medicine formula for their pattern of anxiety would treat both the mental and the physiological component. As they do for disorders of the body, TCM physicians commonly prescribe herbal formulas, acupuncture, and/or moxibustion for mental health conditions—even today, the single most popular herbal formula is one that treats Liver Qi Stagnation, an indication that can include depression and anxiety, as well as irregular bowel movements and irregular menstrual periods. (It is important to keep this in mind and not attempt to use a "one

disease, one treatment" approach, as a single herbal prescription may simultaneously be recommended for a multitude of seemingly unrelated conditions from a Western standpoint.)

In spite of this, there are clearly disorders that are more behavioral than physical, which is what this book will focus on. It is also important to note, even as you navigate through this book, that in addition to treating both mental and physical manifestations of disease, at times a single formula can be used to treat multiple different conditions. This has been summarized in the axiom "one formula, many patterns." Conversely, many

…

terms, such as generalized anxiety disorder or ADHD, can be understood through a similar term in Chinese medicine, such as vexation and agitation, or Running Piglet. Finally, it is worth stressing that physical symptoms, such as those you will read in the charts for each formula, will help you navigate the pattern and formula that best fits you: You might note that you have cold hands and feet and a stitch in your side, and realize this fits the pattern of a specific formula that you find listed under depression. Chinese medicine and this book invite you to pay close attention to your body and mind and the messages it shares with you through your symptoms.

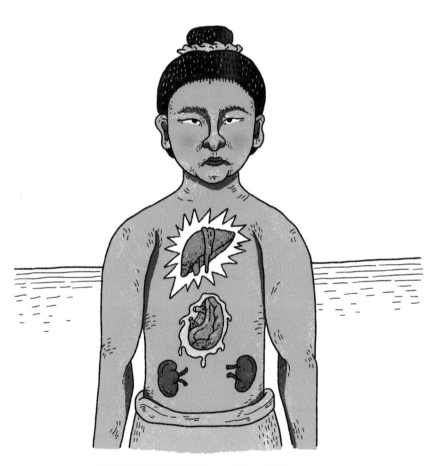

Organ systems referred to in Chinese medicine are not the same as anatomical organs.

Emotions in Chinese Medicine

Emotional and behavioral health have always been key aspects of Chinese medicine. Emotion can even be said to be one of the most direct causes of disease because it is so closely associated with our organs and how they conserve our resources. Have you ever noticed how getting angry produces a powerful rush of energy that ascends and can cause facial flushing, tension in the upper back, and even pain in the side of the body?

If we compare anger to the feeling we would call irritability, we can recognize that it feels similar to anger but is more suppressed and causes a more pervasive feeling of tension and being "stuck," like a bow being pulled back under tension and ready to fire at the least provocation. Both of these patterns are Liver patterns governed by stress and tension; think of it as an irrepressible force meeting an immovable object. In our times, we are faced with so many immovable objects that are overwhelming sources of stress that it is understandable how tensions and frustrations can run high. At the same time, every reaction also has a positive aspect: Resistance to injustice or unfairness can also be a noble expression of the Liver's angry, rising energetic. A sense of direction and strategy is, itself, a sign of a healthy Liver. Chinese medicine has always been an experiential science, investigating what it means to live in the most harmonious and dynamic relationship with one's environment in the broadest possible sense. The factors and forces surrounding us are always in flux, necessarily flowing in some direction.

The Five Phases

Emotions can be categorized according to the Five Phases—Water, Wood, Fire, Earth, and Metal—which are a set of relationships occurring in nature that are a model of change and transformation. The Five Phases is a form of natural science in Chinese culture and philosophy, often used to describe relationships and correspondences between energetic expressions, including from mental to physical to social to cultural and even to political changes or events.

When emotions are viewed through the lens of harmonious function, they are known as Five Emotions (五志). The classics of Chinese medicine recognize the relationship between the Five Emotions and the Five Yin Organs (note, again, that "Organ" here refers to a metaphorical part of a traditional Chinese medical visceral system rather than the actual bodily organ). For example, fear may induce an urge to urinate, which is linked to the Kidney Organ system. This illustrates the fundamental relationship between emotions and health. We can think of this as the movements of the four seasons with an organizing principle. If we think about the movement of the sun, then the four directions are important: the sun rises in the East, reaches its zenith above, descends in the West, and returns to darkness at its lowest point. To observe this, we have to stand on Earth in our bodies—that being the addition that shows the importance of the fifth aspect: Earth itself. Thus, the Five Emotions are ways of looking at our embodied experience.

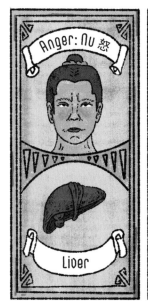
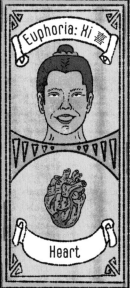
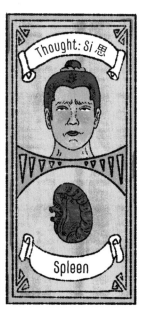
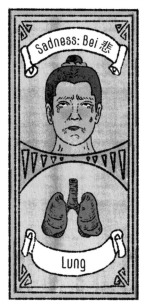
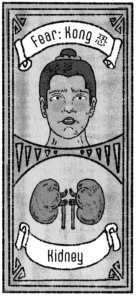

Emotions and their corresponding organs

Let's examine these correspondences:

- North/Water is associated with fear.
- East/Wood is associated with anger.
- South/Fire is associated with joy and excitement.
- Center/Earth is associated with rumination and thought.
- West/Metal is associated with grief and mourning.

We can see how an emotion might be perceived in a sense of tension or rigidity in Wood; excitement or anxiety might be perceived as a flare in the chest; worry might be felt in the pit of the stomach; tearful grief can take one's breath away; and fear can send a shiver down one's spine.

In a similar manner, we can also recognize that certain insults and injuries that affect us resonate with a particular response internally. The loss of a loved one, for example, occasions grief, and grief can produce an oppressive sensation in the chest. The sensation in the chest will make one breathe shallowly. Breathing shallowly creates dysregulation and signals the sympathetic nervous system, causing a stress response. If prolonged, the stress response will produce enervation and fatigue and a diminished immune response, all of which—from the trigger to the body's response to it—represent Lung/Metal factors. We will explore more patterns like this later.

Over time, other emotions were added to the Five Emotions that give us a fuller picture of the body's response to emotion. The clearest expression of emotion as movement is in *Huangdi Neijing* Suwen (Basic Questions), "On Pain":

When one is angry, then the qi rises.
When one is joyous, then the qi relaxes.
When one is sad, then the qi dissipates.
When one is in fear, then the qi moves down.
In case of cold, the qi collects; in case of heat, the qi flows out.
When one is frightened, then the qi is in disorder.
When one is exhausted, then the qi is wasted.
When one is pensive, then the qi lumps together.

Understanding the Effect of Emotion

We have seen that anger makes the qi rise. Let's look at the other emotions to understand their qualities.

Relaxed qi certainly sounds like a good thing, and it is. However, a little too relaxed can describe a state where emotions become a bit too much to handle and even overwhelming.

When one is **sad** and the Lung Organ system is affected, this causes the qi to dissipate. As the Lung is associated with grief, you can imagine what it feels like to lose a loved one, and how loss could be felt as a real sense of emptiness and a lack of vitality.

In fear, which affects the Kidney, there is a sense of collapse, a sense of being so afraid that you curl up into a fetal position (which is even similar to the shape of a kidney). Down and in are similar, so there is an inward retreat in fear.

With **cold and heat**, respectively, we can consider yin and yang. Cold (yin) collects and constricts, and heat (yang) excites and expands outward. Emotionally, this can even mean that cold is something hurtful to you, and heat can be how you lash out from the insult.

Emotion	Organ System	Movement
Anger	Liver	Rising
Joy	Heart	Relaxing, loosening
Sadness	Lung	Dissipating, feeling empty
Fear	Kidney	Descending, retreating
Fright	Heart-Kidney or Bladder	Chaos, panic
Exhaustion	Lung	Depletion, overwhelm
Pensive / Oppression	Spleen	Lumped together, dampening

Fright is like a more yang reaction to fear. This is a startle reaction where energy is mobilized, and one can feel panic or a loss of control. In the experience of Chinese medicine physician Brandt Stickley, this is an important pattern to describe traumatic experience, and the disorder of chaos can imply a separation of form and function (yin and yang)—meaning that emotions are unable to be contained—and creates chaos and vulnerability. When one is exhausted, qi is wasted, meaning that when we are overworked or overwhelmed, or even hypervigilant and overthinking, these conditions are all depleting to the body and mind.

Finally, with **pensiveness**, you might feel like you can't stop thinking about something and your mind keeps going around in circles, causing your qi to clump together and, eventually, lead to a sense of malaise and negativity.

These patterns are a way to help us recognize when our emotions are giving us a message about our circumstances, and perhaps even indicating something we need to change. Acupuncture, acupressure, and herbal medicines help restore a feeling of ease that equips us to care for ourselves and others.

From this basic outline, we can deduce some salient principles governing the Chinese med-icine approach to emotional, mental, and psychological life and well-being. "Psychology" is used here as a term to describe the activity of mind and emotion, which has been noted and observed in Indigenous medicine everywhere since antiquity. Chinese medicine is one such Indigenous system, with the longest and most extensive written traditions available to us. That literary inheritance makes it possible to apply ancient principles to practice today and contributes to the unique position of Chinese medicine to approach contemporary and perennial problems.

The Heart in Chinese Medicine

Keen observation is at the heart of Chinese medicine, and the Heart 心 is central to human life and emotion. The Heart is regarded as the seat of awareness and the mind and, thus, is a core aspect of the self. Since all feelings are processed through awareness, all emotion is ultimately related to the Heart.

What, then, are these Heart-centered principles of Chinese medicine? Emotions are natural phenomena and psychological responses to stimuli. They can be likened to weather patterns or seasonal changes. Our lives and experiences have seasons, and feelings come and go. The first chapter of the *Inner Classic of the Yellow Emperor* informs us of the need to flexibly and dynamically adapt to change, and that when rigidity or habit makes that difficult, problems arise. In modern terms, it is as if all forms of distress are an adjustment disorder. In contrast to conventional medicine, in Chinese medicine, a single symptom or condition is not something we strive to isolate and eliminate. Instead, the medicine works to restore balance among the functions of the body and alleviate suffering as a result.

We are not all endowed with the same resources, and we are certainly not all the same. Our terrain may be weathered by our experience, body condition, and circumstances—some adverse and some advantageous. But we can each be met as we are and accorded respect for our very being. This illustrates the nonpathologizing potential within traditional models.

Our reactions to stress are all creative ways of adapting to differing circumstances, and this is true of immediate emotional reactions and enduring aspects of personality. The expressions of the Five Phases are true at all scales in space and time—where we are and where we are going, across days, months, seasons, years, decades, lifetimes.

Conclusion

After reading chapter 2, you may have a better understanding of the relationship between phases, emotions, and even direction. These ancient concepts have been cornerstones of this rich medical tradition for millennia and further emphasize the connection between our mind and body. Symptoms, both physical and emotional, are messages serving our becoming. Just as we are embedded within a terrain, we are also always in relationship to other beings, events, and things, and our lives are expressions of the ways that we make contact with those forces in an attempt to stay in touch with our inner resources.

In the following chapter, you will learn about the various healing modalities within traditional Chinese medicine, particularly herbal medicine. We explore why multi-herb formulas are used almost exclusively and what toxicity means in a TCM context. You will also learn about Five Element music therapy, the principles of Chinese medicine food therapy, and qigong, as well as some common causes of disharmony, and be introduced to the concept of yangsheng, or self-cultivation.

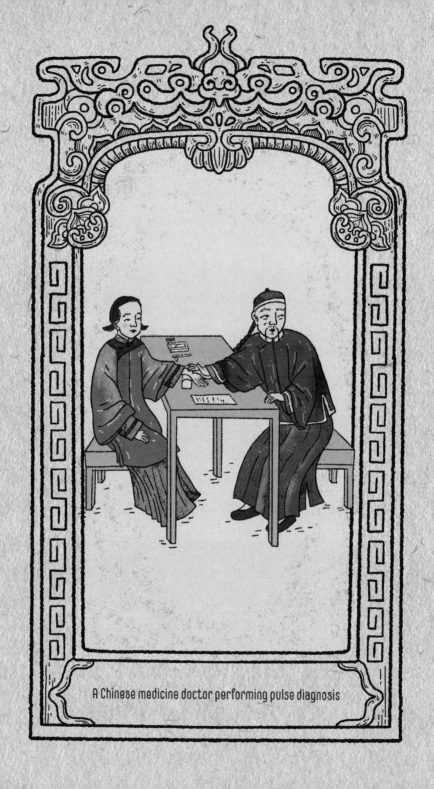

A Chinese medicine doctor performing pulse diagnosis

Chapter 3

TRADITIONAL CHINESE MEDICINE'S HEALING MODALITIES

The average person in the West likely thinks of acupuncture as the quintessential traditional Chinese medicine healing method. However, to the average person in China, acupuncture often takes a back seat to herbal formulas, which are generally considered the go-to TCM healing modality and often thought to be more effective than acupuncture for a wider range of conditions. Furthermore, moxibustion is just as popular as acupuncture, and perhaps even more frequently performed because people can easily do it themselves. Doctors skilled at prescribing herbal formulas are also generally thought to occupy a more prestigious role in Chinese society compared to acupuncturists. (Unfortunately, herbal formulas are not a required part of the curriculum of most Chinese medicine schools in the United States, and only a small percent of acupuncturists in the United States have herbal medicine training.) If you're looking to continue your journey with Chinese medicine, we recommend seeking licensed acupuncturists who have training in herbal medicine.

Here are some of the more popular healing modalities in Chinese medicine that will be featured in this book.

Chinese Herbal Formulas

Chinese herbal formulas are the Chinese medicine equivalent of medications or supplements. These medicines are called "herbal formulas" because they comprise multiple herbs—unlike Western herbalism, Chinese medicine almost never recommends single herbs as medicines for reasons explained further on in this chapter, instead favoring what are known as complex synergistic or compound formulas. (Note: The term "herb" in a traditional Chinese medicine context does not have the same meaning as "herb" in a Western sense. In Chinese medicine, herbs include various plants, mushrooms, minerals, medicinal foods, and any other ingredients that would be used as medicine. Beef collagen and egg yolk are two ingredients you'll find in an herbal formula in this book.)

Using Chinese Herbal Formulas

One of the biggest surprises for me when I launched my company, The Eastern Philosophy, was the unexpectedly large proportion of people assuming all herbal medicine came only in "tea" form. Chinese herbal medicine taken orally comes in a variety of prepared formats, including small round pills, boluses (chewable herbal balls), tablets, granules, powders, tinctures, and more.

The most well-known TCM format is a decoction, which is made by boiling raw herbs in water and then simmering them, usually for about an hour. Although some may colloquially refer to this as "tea," the Chinese term for decoction is tang (汤), meaning "soup," which more accurately describes the cooking process. Decoctions are sometimes prescribed by practitioners but have decreased in popularity due to the time-consuming process needed to create them.

Although it may be tempting and comforting to find raw herbs yourself to make these formulas, I do not recommend this for a number of reasons:

- TCM herbs exist in different preparations with distinct properties, which can be quite difficult to identify and confirm.

- The quality of imported raw herbs in stores often varies, and in general, is not as high quality as those used in prepared herbal medicine formulas.

- Herbs grown in different regions often have a wide range of pharmacological activity, which can make certain origins or herbs more or less suitable for certain formulas.

If, however, you are decocting herbs at home, it is important to know that herbal formulas should always be taken in their complete form and as indicated—and not revised, with specific herbs added or removed—unless under the guidance of a practitioner who has assessed your condition. Certain individual herbs within a compound formula may have pharmacological properties or toxicities that are amplified, reduced, or negated by the addition of another herb. Furthermore, newcomers to TCM often ask only for the ingredients of various herbal formulas without realizing that just as crucial as the list of ingredients is the *ratio* of each herb in the overall formula, as well as the overall dosage. Formulas are delicately, painstakingly calibrated and balanced in a way that makes dosages absolutely critical to their efficacy and reduction of side effects. *Herbs should not be purchased and haphazardly prepared on your own.*

For the purposes of both accessibility and safety, most of the formulas in the book are available as "patent formulas." Here, "patent" alludes to standardization, not legal rights. Chinese patent medicines are the equivalent of generic, over-the-counter medicines and are available in ready-to-use formats such as pills, tablets, and granules. Reputable patent medicine manufacturers following Good Agricultural Practices (GAP) and Good Manufacturing Practices (GMP) monitor botanical identification, collection, post-harvest processing, and agriculture contaminants, including heavy metals, pesticides, fungicides, herbicides, and bacteria, plant, and fungal contaminants.

How to Take Chinese Herbal Formulas

Most Chinese herbal medicine should be taken with warm water and should simply be swallowed, not dissolved. This includes round pills (wan), which are likely the most popular format of Chinese medicine and are colloquially known as "tea pills." Do not take herbal medicine with beverages other than water, especially juice or coffee. These can

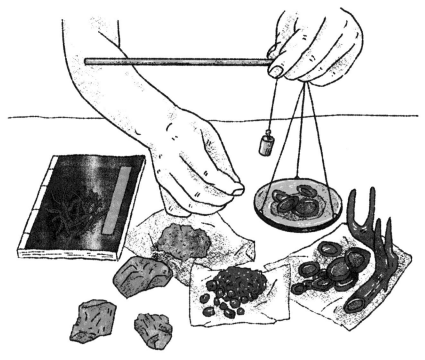

An assortment of non-botanical herbs, including minerals, deer antler, and cordyceps

have an effect on the pharmacological activity of the herbs, an effect that is also recognized in Western biomedicine: According to a 2021 review, "Fruit juices contain a large number of phytochemicals that, in combination with certain drugs, can cause food-drug interactions that can be clinically significant and lead to adverse events." Similarly, several studies and medical case reports show that concomitant consumption of coffee significantly affects the absorption, distribution, metabolism, and excretion of many drugs. This is also why trendy mushroom coffees are not recommended from a TCM perspective! Most TCM herbal formulas—unless specified—are also fine to take while

on Western medications if spaced out by at least one hour.

When reading the Chinese name of an herbal formula, the last word typically denotes the dosage form of the medicine. For example, Bu Nao Wan and Bu Nao Pian are the same formula, but one comes in round pills (wan) whereas the other comes in tablets (pian). Unless specified, you may take an herbal formula for four to six weeks at full dosage, after which you can reduce the dosage, take as needed, or stop taking. Most people will notice a difference within the first week of starting the formula. If you notice no difference, it may not be the right formula for you.

Lastly, I recommend avoiding websites such as Amazon when you purchase Chinese medicine because they have been known to carry counterfeit products.

Complex Herbal Formulas in Traditional Chinese Medicine, Not Single Ingredients

One of the most confusing aspects of Chinese medicine to those accustomed to Western biomedicine, or even Western herbalism, is the fact that so many herbs are used in one Chinese medicine formula. Questions frequently include some variant of, "What's the active ingredient so I can just take that?" or "Why don't they just isolate the compound?" These demonstrate a conventional Western medicine approach to a different medical system that goes against one of the most beneficial and unique aspects of Chinese herbal medicine.

TCM formulas have at least two herbs, and sometimes upward of ten herbs or more, to enhance the bioavailability of the active herb, promote therapeutic effects, and reduce side effects, with a result that is synergistic and much greater than the sum of its parts. These compound, or complex synergistic formulas, are also able to address multiple causes of disease. As already noted, Western medicine has usually relied on a "one drug, one target" approach. However, many studies have demonstrated that multiple herbs in complex formulations offer better efficacies than equivalent doses of individual active ingredients/herbs, highlighting the significance of synergistic action in herbal medicine. Synthetic mono-drugs have been increasingly found to have more side effects, limited effectiveness in chronic diseases, and treatment resistance.

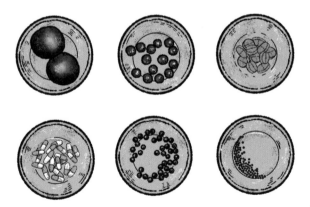

Various TCM dosage forms, including wan, honey boluses, pian, and capsules

Chinese medicine formula architecture follows the Jun-Chen-Zuo-Shi 君-臣-佐-使, or Emperor-Minister-Assistant-Courier, model to achieve desired medicinal effects and to minimize side effects, with each nonleading herb having a specific role to serve the leading Jun/Emperor herb:

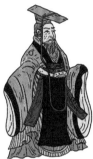

Jun/Emperor 君

The Jun/Emperor is the *main herb or herbs* in an herbal formula with a relatively higher ratio directly targeting the disease.

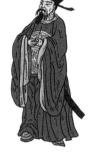

Chen/Minister 臣

The Chen/Minister is an *adjuvant herb*— one that promotes the therapeutic effect of the main herb or targets accompanying symptoms.

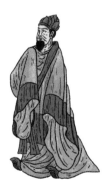

Zuo/Assistant 佐

The Zuo/Assistant is usually used to *reduce side effects*

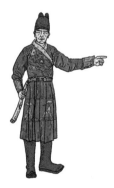

Shi/Courier 使

The Shi/Courier *guides the active ingredients* to reach the target Organs or to harmonize their actions.

In Chinese herbal medicine, well-balanced formulas are those designed to fully anticipate possible adverse side effects and preemptively resolve them by adding specific herbs within the formula. With few exceptions, *this book focuses on well-balanced formulas with low or no toxicity that are widely available, and includes the function of each herb in the formula and the symptoms they respectively treat*

A Note on Toxicity

Just as many common over-the-counter (OTC) products in Western medicine have known toxicity, such as acetaminophen (Tylenol), certain herbs used in Chinese medicine may also have some level of toxicity. This is often mitigated within a formula, prepared in a way to minimize the adverse effects, or taken only for limited amounts of time for a specific condition. In certain cases, these herbs are "borrowed" and incorporated into the West improperly, resulting in serious side effects, as summarized by one research article: "The main impediment for the introduction of TCM in the Western world is not the lack of evidence on the efficacy, but reports on its toxicity caused by its incorrect use." An example of this is Ma Huang, an herb that has been used for thousands of years in Chinese medicine. Considered one of the most effective medicinals for respiratory conditions such as asthma due to its broncho-dilating properties, Ma Huang was known to have some toxicity and so was only prescribed short term in multi-herb formulas.

Unfortunately, Ma Huang was "adopted" in the West and marketed by unscrupulous companies as the performance-enhancing or weight loss supplement called Ephedra.

This resulted in numerous reports of serious cardiovascular side effects, and the U.S. Food and Drug Administration (FDA) issued regulations prohibiting the sale of all supplements containing Ephedra, as well as TCM formulas containing Ma Huang. However, this ruling was based primarily on the misuse of Ma Huang: Ephedra was administered in isolation and at a relatively high dose as a slimming agent, indicating an incorrect use of a Chinese medicine herb. Incidents like this have given TCM a bad reputation for using herbs deemed toxic or dangerous, thus hampering the introduction of TCM in the West. It's also worth keeping in mind that one of the most toxic drugs is acetaminophen (Tylenol): It results in 56,000 emergency department visits per year and is the number-one cause of liver transplantation in the United States. However, at recommended doses, acetaminophen is considered to have a good safety profile.

Mercurials, or substances containing mercury, are also occasionally and selectively used in Eastern medicine, including traditional Chinese medicine and Ayurveda—a fact that uninformed people may point to as proof of TCM's "antiquated" nature. Arsenic is both a poison and a medicine, documented in numerous classical Chinese medicine texts as a substance with "great toxicity," yet under certain conditions, it is considered an appropriate medicine. One of these conditions is acute promyelocytic leukemia, which was one of the most aggressive and fatal forms of acute leukemia but which has now become one of the most treatable forms, with an 80 percent cure rate. The reason for this is a treatment directly borrowed from traditional Chinese medicine: arsenic trioxide. After scientists in China in the 1970s discovered its effectiveness in treating acute promyelocytic leukemia, a series of clinical trials in the United States confirmed the findings, and arsenic trioxide was approved by the FDA in 2000 as a treatment. One of the doctors who led some of the National Institutes of Health–funded studies published a research article in *Expert Review of Anticancer Therapy* concluding that in the context of acute promyelocytic leukemia, arsenic trioxide is "definitely not a poison; the data suggest that it is more of a magic potion." However, it is only used in specific cases.

Acupuncture

Acupuncture is one of the simplest healing instruments, performed using a stainless-steel needle inserted strategically into various acupuncture points of the body—specific anatomic points on the body that have been shown to treat a variety of health issues through stimulation. In the West, acupuncture is often incorrectly believed to primarily treat pain or musculoskeletal issues and, although studies show it is effective for both pain and injuries, acupuncture can actually be used in the treatment of most conditions, including mental health issues. In fact, one of the most well-known protocols in acupuncture is used to relieve severe mental health disorders.

In Neolithic times, acupuncture needles were made of Bian stone, animal bone, and horn, and later made with metals such as bronze and gold; steel needles were used in China starting around 300 CE. Acupuncture is close to becoming mainstream in North America—it's covered by Medicaid and many health insurance plans for certain conditions, and some hospitals provide acupuncture services as part of their integrative medicine and oncology departments. Although researchers are still theorizing about specific mechanisms of action, there have been numerous placebo-controlled studies on acupuncture dating back to the 1960s. Contemporary medical research shows that acupuncture regulates the immune system, reduces inflammation, and boosts nutrients in the blood, which help cells repair and heal. There is also growing clinical evidence of acupuncture's effects on mental health, including a 2021 study that showed it can reduce anxiety, and a 2020 systematic review found it was more effective in treating chronic pain with depression than prescription medication.

Acupressure and Moxibustion

These two healing methods use the same theories as acupuncture—targeting acupoints on the body and stimulating them by either applying pressure (acupressure) or holding a burning moxibustion stick close to the acupoint (moxibustion). Moxibustion involves burning the herb mugwort (usually rolled into in a stick or "cigar"), which we burn to emit targeted heat at the acupoints, instead of stimulating these acupoints with needles. Although moxibustion is relatively unknown in the West, it is just as popular as acupuncture in China, especially because it is often performed at home. Since this book focuses on at-home remedies, a number of exercises refer to acupressure, but moxibustion can be performed instead. If you live in an apartment, use smokeless moxibustion sticks, made of mugwort charcoal, as regular moxibustion sticks emit a very strong smoke and smell.

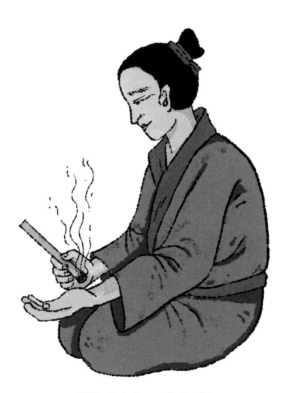

A TCM patient using a moxibustion stick

Five Element Music Therapy

Of all the time-tested healing modalities in traditional Chinese medicine, the one that happens to be among the least known in the West is a musical prescription: Five Element music therapy. First defined in the *Book of Rites*, a collection of texts describing society and rituals of the Zhou dynasty (1046–256 BCE) and compiled from 51 to 21 BCE, Five Element music therapy combines the theory of the five elements (Wood, Fire, Earth, Metal, Water) with the Chinese five-note (pentatonic) scale to treat mind-body disorders. It is performed on classical Chinese musical instruments such as the dizi, erhu, guqin, pipa, and zither. It's also a healing remedy that is uniquely accessible and safe, which has made it a popular therapy in recent years for seniors, pregnant people, and cancer patients.

The ancient Chinese identified the healing properties of music long ago: The traditional characters for music (樂) and medicine (藥) are nearly identical and transform to medicine only by adding a small grass "radical" on top of the character for music. Dating back to prehistoric shamanic traditions, this type of music therapy was subsequently documented in China's first medical text, *Inner Classic of the Yellow Emperor*. The ancient Chinese chose five notes to make up their classical musical scale—Gong (do in the Western scale), Shang (re), Jue (mi), Zhi (so), Yu (la)—each one corresponding to an element in the Five Element theory: Earth, Metal, Wood, Fire, and Water, respectively. These elements are also foundational to the TCM Organ system, and each musical note in the traditional Chinese pentatonic scale was believed to correspond to an Organ system. Thus, music of a certain key has its own distinct qualities.

This notion of each scale possessing different qualities is not unique to Chinese music; a parallel concept in Western music is the Greek modes, which also have moods and characteristics unique to each mode due to the intervals of the notes. For example, Lydian is considered dreamy and mysterious, Phrygian is dark and exotic. However, unlike Western music, Chinese Five Element music is theorized to nourish and reach harmonious resonance with each corresponding Organ system, thus healing specific ailments, including disorders of the mind.

Five Element Music Therapy: Pentatonic Scale

Note	Pitch	Western Scale Syllable	Element	Organ System
Gong	C	do	Earth	Spleen
Shang	D	re	Metal	Lung
Jue	E	mi	Wood	Liver
Zhi	G	sol	Fire	Heart
Yu	A	la	Water	Kidney

Five Element music is deeply inspired by nature and has an idyllic, pastoral quality that first-time listeners often describe as "relaxing" or "peaceful." Increasing research has shown that listening to this ancient music can significantly alter both physical and mental health. Studies show it can reduce insomnia, depression, and anxiety; treat seasonal affective disorder; and improve quality of life. A 2020 meta-analysis even showed that it can significantly improve labor pain and duration and reduce hemorrhaging in perinatal women. Although this type of music dates back to ancient times, modern music therapy in China is quite recent, originating in 1979. However, after the first music therapy department was created at Changsha Sanatorium in 1984, a study was released detailing a new music therapy treatment model, which was widely covered by mainstream newspapers, ushering the field of Chinese music therapy into an era of rapid development and interest.

Before skeptics point to cultural bias in the studies, a group of scientists decided to test the effects of different types of music at the cellular level—and the extraordinary findings could convince even the most dedicated rock devotee to rethink their playlists! The researchers played three different types of music to in vitro embryonic kidney cells: Five Element music, Western classical, and rock. The results were astounding. Unlike rock and classical music, exposing human cells to Five Element music produced several beneficial physiological effects, including statistically significant increases in the production of ATP (which can increase energy and boost cognitive function) by 17 percent and glutathione (which helps prevent cellular damage and modulates inflammatory response) by 21 percent, as well as a significant reduc-

tion in reactive oxygen species (indicating decreased oxidative stress) by 13 percent. Furthermore, while classical music resulted in flat or less notable physiological effects, in sharp contrast, cells treated with heavy metal music showed significant oxidative stress. These study findings indicate that listening to Five Element music has significant effects on healing both body and mind.

To benefit from Five Element music therapy, you don't need to listen to this type of music all day long or at the exclusion of everything else. Participants in studies listened to Five Element music anywhere from one to two hours per week to two hours a day. If you're new to this genre, you can check out our playlist—The Eastern Philosophy's Picks: 5ElementMusic—on Spotify or search for tried-and-true classics (see chapter 4, Insomnia, and chapter 6, Anxiety, which recommend specific tracks by name). Note that while many versions of these musical classics exist, including versions with vocals or played by Western orchestras, the most beneficial therapeutically are likely those using only classic Chinese instruments.

Food Therapy

Food as medicine is a core tenet of Chinese culture, an idea encapsulated in the expression "yao shi tong yuan" (药食同源), meaning food and medicine have the same source. Traditional Chinese cuisine is extremely thoughtful in its approach to food, and what we eat is considered paramount to both physical and mental health in Chinese medicine.

According to multiple studies, the shift away from traditional lifestyles has been linked to increased rates of depression and other mental health disorders—which some academics have dubbed "diseases of modernity"—and increasingly, studies have demonstrated the protective effects of a traditional diet against mental health disorders, depression in particular. Mental health disorders are often characterized by chronic, low-grade inflammation and oxidative stress, and the gut microbiome can contribute to altered mood. Unfortunately, an inflammatory microbiome can, at least, be partially linked to common Western dietary habits.

Healthy eating in Chinese medicine terms has a different meaning than it does in the West: A smoothie for breakfast and a salad for lunch would likely be considered healthy choices in the West, but from a TCM perspective, overloading one's body with raw, cold food and drink can be harmful to health, and over time, can be one of the leading external causes of imbalance and disease. Younger women are considered particularly susceptible to Dampness (more on this in later chapters) due to lifestyle habits that often involve consuming cold food and drink, along with overworking or overexercising.

Furthermore, trendy "healthy" eating in the West often consists of extreme diets, such as juicing, raw paleo, or keto, with potential negative longer-term consequences. Studies on both humans and mice show that keto diets lead to decreased levels of Bifidobacterium, lowering microbiome diversity, which is linked to ulcerative colitis and inflammatory bowel disease.

In contrast, Chinese medicine wisdom emphasizes the idea of balance in the diet—according to the Suwen section of the *Huangdi Neijing*, we should take grains to nourish, fruit to assist, livestock to benefit, and vegetables to supplement. Even the traditional communal style of Chinese eating, in which family and friends share dishes around the table, emphasizes an element of diversity and balance of multiple ingredients, food groups, and flavors.

Similar to the TCM approach to medicinal herbs, food ingredients can also be cooling or warming (as well as cold, hot, or mild), terms that describe the effect they have on our bodies. While the "cooling or heating" nature of foods seems to be a point that Westerners, or even younger generations of Chinese, think of as mere superstitions, some are beginning to be validated by scientific studies. Take ginger, for example—one of the foods (and herbs) in TCM most recognized for its warming properties, commonly recommended to people with poor circulation or cold hands and feet. A team of Japanese researchers designed a placebo-controlled crossover trial and measured the palm temperatures of women with cold-sensitive extremities, discovering that increased palm temperature following ginger intake was maintained significantly longer than after placebo intake.

The following are the core principles of healthy eating, according to traditional Chinese medicine and cuisine:

1. Avoid food and drink that are cold in temperature, especially iced drinks.

2. Eat cooked foods; fruit is an exception.

3. Try to eat foods that fall into all flavors: sweet, sour, bitter, salty, pungent/spicy.

4. Eat fermented foods often: Food fermentation is extremely prevalent in East Asian food and beverage culture, including fermented soy milk, jiu niang (酒釀) (fermented sweet rice), kimchi, kombucha, miso, pu'er tea, and red yeast rice. The fermentation process can improve the digestibility of nutrients in products of plant origin and boosts the bioavailability of nutrients—fermenting rice overnight increases iron content by as much as twenty-one times! Fermented foods also alter your gut microbiome, leading to lower levels of inflammation.

5. Avoid overly rich and ultra-processed foods.

6. Eat more mushrooms: Mushrooms are highly popular in Asian cuisine, and new evidence indicates they benefit mental health. A study from Pennsylvania State University's School of Medicine on mushroom intake and depression found that eating mushrooms was associated with lower rates of depression. According to the lead researcher, mushrooms are the highest dietary source of ergothioneine, an anti-inflammatory amino acid that may lower the risk of oxidative stress, which could also reduce the symptoms of depression.

Qigong

Qigong comprises mind-body exercises with roots in Chinese medicine and philosophy, used for the purpose of both physical and mental health. The physical exercises are often considered a form of dynamic meditation.

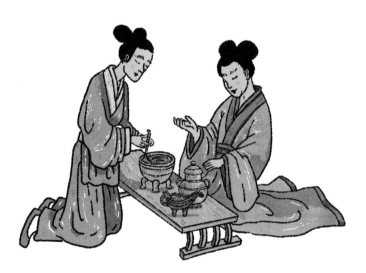

The preparation of herbal soup

Interview with Daniel Spigelman

Q: What is qigong, and what was the purpose behind its creation?

A: The term "qigong" (氣功) literally means "work with qi," or "qi skill," and encompasses not only breathing exercises but also visualization and meditative practices, self-massage, stretching, gymnastic routines with an emphasis on posture similar to some elements of yoga, as well as other more esoteric pursuits. Such practices have a long history in ancient China dating back to at least the Warring States Period (475–221 BCE), possibly far older, with roots in shamanic practice. However, "qigong" is a relatively modern term, commonly used starting in the 1950s. These types of exercises were historically practiced to cure disease and assist in increasing health, vitality, and longevity as well as for more arcane, spiritual purposes, including communion with cosmic deities and achieving immortality.

Q: What is the difference between the various forms of qigong?
What is qigong versus tai chi?

A: A multitude of different qigong systems exist, some attached to specific religious or spiritual beliefs, or schools of philosophy, most notably Daoism, Confucianism, and Buddhism. There are medical systems of qigong, some designed to assist patients in their recovery from illness, others with the intention of developing the capacities of the healer to treat diseases. There are also martial systems of qigong with aims of conditioning the body for combat. Many of the training exercises of Taiji quan (太極拳) (tai chi), originally created as a martial art, would fit into this category, although there is often overlap between the martial and medical, with tai chi often being lauded for its health benefits. Folk systems of qigong also exist that do not fit neatly into any of the aforementioned categories.

Q: What is the theory behind how qigong can improve psychological
and emotional well-being?

A: Three major principles found in qigong practices are Adjusting One's Heart-Mind (調心), Adjusting One's Breathing (調息), and Adjusting One's Physical Structure (調形), with all three able to influence mental health positively. Depending on the specific practice, focus can be on one, two, or all three of these elements. These elements are not completely disparate and share a significant degree of mutual influence. Physical posture, especially the holding of tension, and habitual breathing patterns can both have a noticeable effect on mental health. The Heart is seen as the seat of emotions in traditional Chinese thought and, as such, practices involving the Heart-Mind can help improve mental health issues, including ADHD, anxiety, autism, and depression. Qigong practiced over time will develop focus, calm the mind, provide tools for everyday emotional regulation, improve posture, and boost vascular and neurological function. Many of these mental health issues are broadly diagnosed as "stagnation syndrome" (鬱症) in traditional Chinese medicine. We know from classic Chinese medical texts that there is a long history of emotional irregularities causing a congestion of qi, which can in turn manifest in a variety of different further symptoms and disease classifications. Regular qigong practice can help such diagnoses by unblocking and moving qi.

It should be firmly stated, however, that there are risks involved in unsupervised qigong practice, especially in those with mental health issues. Those with severe mental health issues or a family history of such should not practice unless being guided by an experienced teacher, as improper execution of techniques may cause unwanted side effects and exacerbate these conditions. If symptoms worsen as a result of practice, one should stop immediately and seek treatment from a trained professional.

Yangsheng (養生) (Nourishing Life)

While wellness has become increasingly mainstream over the past decade, it has a long history in ancient Chinese culture. Yangsheng devotees have been obsessed with the concept of wellness and self-cultivation since at least the Han dynasty (202–220 CE). Yangsheng practices include mind-body exercises, breathwork, self-massage, fasting, sexual practices, herbal medicine, food therapy, and, in extreme cases, even alchemy—all in an effort to proactively improve health and prolong life.

Interview with Z'ev Rosenberg

Z'ev Rosenberg, LAc, practitioner, educator, and author of three books, including Returning to the Source, *is recognized as one of the first generation of practitioners of traditional Chinese medicine in America. He was one of the initiators of an acupuncture licensing law in Colorado. As well as being professor and chair emeritus at Pacific College of Health and Science, he has lectured widely around the United States and serves as a professor at the Academy of Chinese Culture and Health Sciences in Oakland, California, and Five Branches Institute in San Jose, California.*

Q: You're considered an expert on yangsheng in the United States. How did you end up getting interested in this topic?

A: My interest in yangsheng stems from my teens, when, due to poor respiratory health growing up in the polluted, damp, and cold environment of New York, I was seeking better health. When I was seventeen years old, I discovered macrobiotics through an interview with John Lennon, and I was eating in macrobiotic restaurants in the East Village of Manhattan before attending concerts at the Fillmore East. As it turns out, macrobiotics was based on yin/yang and Five Phase theory, which led to my interest in Asian medical systems. Interestingly, Paul Unschuld, in his *Medicine in China* series, translated yangsheng as "macrobiotics," and certainly that was the intention of that school of thought, even though it was somewhat removed from its roots in the Han dynasty medical canon.

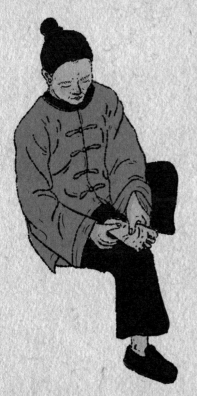

Q: People in the West use the term "self-care," which has become a wellness trend. How would you explain yangsheng to someone who practices self-care but is new to Chinese medicine?

A: I don't find that wellness trends in the West are clearly defined in terms of guiding principles; they tend to be empirical findings of different methods and ideas, often still maintaining a Western biomedical or naturopathic perspective. Asian medicine has

A person administering
self-massage

45

its roots in natural law, based on the *Yi Jing*'s understanding of cycles and transformations. So one is teaching a philosophy of life first and foremost. Then, one can look at techniques, whether Eastern or Western in origin.

Q: You have written that "the vast system of Chinese/Asian medicine in its foundation is about preserving, nurturing, and maintaining health, and only secondarily about treating disease." These may be new approaches to health for many people who are accustomed to Western medicine's treatment-focused approach. Why do you think these concepts within Chinese medicine are striking a chord with so many people today?

A: There comes a point in a culture of excess when a desire for simplicity and grounding returns. There are only so many procedures, surgeries, and/or medications a person can take and, before long, they start producing iatrogenic effects. More and more, people are open to simplicity, managing their own health and finding new solutions. This is compounded by the insane costs of medical care and medications in the United States, the dead ends of such regimens as Ozempic for weight loss, and the fact that the ER is the first-line doctor's office for so many people now. Many doctors have a six-month or more waiting list to see them.

Q: What yangsheng practices, medicinals, or habits would you recommend to support general mental health, or alleviate issues such as anxiety, brain fog, depression, insomnia, or trauma?

A: This is a broad question and the answer, of course, must be tailored to an individual's needs, season, age group, sex, and personality. That said, certainly regulating sleep, meditation/prayer, therapeutic exercise, eating a plant-based diet—which does not necessarily mean vegan or vegetarian—with fermented foods, and medicinal mushrooms can be recommended for almost everyone.

Q: Are there any yangsheng practices, medicinals, or habits you think are crucial for everyone?

A: Qigong or yoga, walking in nature (forest bathing), hot springs, therapeutic baths with bath salts and aromatherapy oils, quality sleep, healthy family relationships, diet that is as local and organic as possible, miso soup, fermented vegetables, and medicinal mushrooms such as lingzhi/reishi, Cordyceps, lion's mane, and chaga. In addition, regular acupuncture/moxibustion and herbal medicine, which can also support health as well as treat illnesses by regulating the channel system, the true genius of the Chinese medical tradition. As Zhang Xichun said, "Acumoxa and herbal medicine are tools to teach our patients the philosophy of the *Neijing*."

Conclusion

You should now have a good understanding of some of the healing modalities within Chinese medicine, including food and music therapy, as well as why complex, synergistic herbal formulas are used instead of just a single ingredient. You were also introduced to qigong and yangsheng—the ancient practice of self-cultivation—from two experts.

The subsequent six chapters focus on common mental health conditions, with insight into the history, clinical approach, and patterns as well as herbal formulas and a variety of other Chinese medicine therapies to address these conditions.

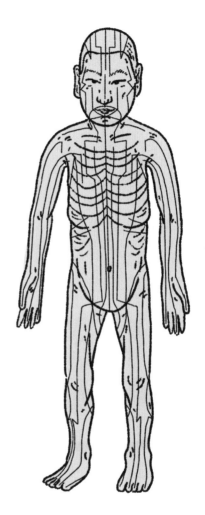

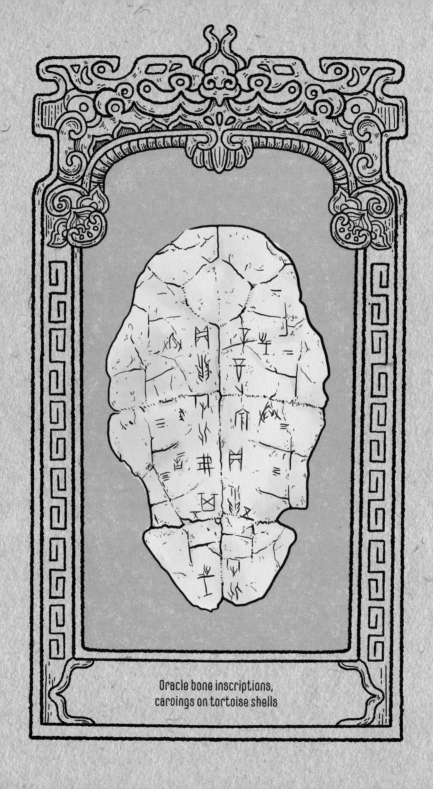

Oracle bone inscriptions,
carvings on tortoise shells

CHAPTER 4

INSOMNIA

In Chinese medicine, sleep has long been considered the most significant influence on our health and is often an expression of emotional tension. Physicians throughout ancient China created detailed roadmaps for sleep hygiene, from bi-hourly body clocks recommending optimal sleep times to herbal formulas to target a diverse range of sleep disturbances. Technology developed to relax the mind and body and encourage high-quality sleep were so common throughout ancient China that we can find these artifacts in major museums today: hard pillows made of jade or ceramic stimulated acupoints along the back of the head to activate the parasympathetic nervous system. There are even acupoints named after these pillows: sustained pressure on the Yuzhen (玉枕), or Jade Pillow points, help release neck and shoulder tension. We will explore many of these time-tested techniques for sleep throughout this chapter, including acupressure and qigong exercises, foot soaks, tui na massage, Five Element music therapy, and, of course, herbal medicine.

The term "insomnia" can refer to a variety of disturbances relating to sleep, including difficulty falling asleep, waking up several times during the night, lying awake at night, and other symptoms indicating poor quality of sleep. The *Inner Classic of the Yellow Emperor* details how sleep initiates when qi and blood circulating on the surface of the body flow inward, gathering in the Organs. If a blockage occurs, either due to external or internal influences, this flow cannot move inward, preventing sleep from initiating. This concept is summarized as "yang cannot enter yin."

This ancient concept is remarkably similar to our modern understanding of sleep: Research shows that alterations to the body's circulation that occur as we prepare for sleep affect core temperature, a major trigger for sleep initiation. Sleep expert Saul Gilbet and colleagues found that surface blood circulation peaks as a person prepares to go to sleep and then gathers into the organs

once sleep has initiated. This drop in core temperature is thought to trigger the onset of sleep.

While some traditional Chinese medicine formulas for sleep include sedative herbs, the main focus is to restore the normal circadian flow of qi and blood through the body. These herbal formulas for insomnia may not provide the groggy, sedating feeling of Western sleep drugs, but they help restore the body's natural rhythm and internal signaling, which allows the sleep-wake cycle to reset naturally.

An Historian's Overview of Insomnia in Traditional Chinese Medicine

References to sleep date back as far as the oldest records of writing in ancient China. The oracle bone script, the earliest form of Chinese writing, already contains extensive records of sleep and dreams. Dream interpretation was a key feature in the earliest Chinese medical classic, *Inner Classic of the Yellow Emperor*. Based on the theories of qi, yin-yang, and the Five Phases, the *Inner Classic* suggests that different dreams are indicative of different states of qi. For example, dreaming of flying indicates an abundance of qi above (in the upper body), while dreaming of falling suggests an abundance of qi below (in the lower body). Dreams of anger are associated with an abundance of Liver Qi, whereas dreams of weeping are linked to an abundance of Lung Qi. The *Inner Classic* also emphasizes that an uncomfortable stomach is the key reason for an uncomfortable sleep.

In Zhang Zhongjing's classic medical text, *Shanghanlun*, sleep disorders were categorized into patterns based on pathologies. This text recommended different remedies for various types of insomnia on the basis of pattern differentiation.

For **Greater Yang insomnia**, characterized by feelings of unease and listlessness in the Heart accompanied by unquiet sleep, Gardenia and Fermented Soybean Decoction (see page 60) was suggested.

For **Lesser Yin insomnia**, marked by vexation in the Heart and inability to sleep, Coptis and E Jiao Decoction (see page 58) was proposed.

For **sleeplessness** caused by blood impediment and vacancy taxation, Sour Jujube Seed Decoction (see page 56) was recommended.

To treat **restless legs syndrome** during nighttime, *Shanghanlun* recommended Peony and Licorice Decoction.

These remedies continue to be used widely by Chinese medical practitioners in treating sleep disorders.

The correlation between emotional disorders and sleep disorders was recognized in the tenth century. The *Peaceful Holy Benevolent Prescriptions* regarded the cause of insomnia to be Heart vacuity, with signs of a feeling of emptiness in the Heart and susceptibility to fright and fear. In Chinese medicine, the "spirit" (shen 神) is believed to be stored in the Heart. If the Heart fails to govern the spirit, it will result in sleep disorders or nightmares secondary to emotional disorders.

Since the fifteenth century, the primary understanding of insomnia has been based on the breakdown of the Heart-Kidney interaction—a disorder of the normal relationship between Heart yang and Kidney yin. The Heart yang is likened to heaven and the sun, and if the sun were to lose its location, the spirit qi would drift around. The Kidney yin is like Earth and Water. Under the bright sun, Water in Earth rises and turns into clouds and the qi of Heart yang; clouds, originating from the Heart yang, nourish the Kidney yin. This is how the Heart and Kidney interact in the human body. Remedies for noninteraction of the Heart and Kidney insomnia include herbal formulas such as Heart-Kidney Pills and Peaceful Interaction Pills, acupuncture, and meditation to supplement the Kidney and drain the Heart.

Chinese medicine employs these natural remedies to restore the balance and connection between yin and yang, Liver and Lung, and Heart and Kidney. Once the body and mind are in harmony, the natural cycle and quality of sleep will be restored.

A Clinician's Approach to Insomnia in Traditional Chinese Medicine

Patterns of rest and activity are of paramount importance in Chinese medicine. Wen Zhi, a famous Warring States Period (475–221 BCE) physician, declared, "I give priority to sleep ... it is the first thing for health preservation." Similarly, the first chapter of the *Inner Classic of the Yellow Emperor* stresses that insufficient rest and recovery lead to distress and decrease life span. There are multiple terms applied to insomnia in classical Chinese medical literature that describe degrees of severity, from an inability to sleep all the way to an inability to even lie down.

As just stated, the most fundamental issue pertaining to sleep is the ability of the Heart to settle into a quiet state. A line in Zhang Zhongjing's *Shanghanlun* connects an inability to sleep with "an anguish in the heart, hard to articulate." In traditional Chinese medical terms, this is described as "yang descending into yin." In Organ terms, the Heart and Kidney axis are of primary importance.

All of these terms have significant overlapping concepts, including circadian rhythm, sleep hygiene, internal temperature changes facilitating or inhibiting sleep, and hormones such as melatonin and cortisol. But even complex physiological relationships can still be understood through the dynamics of yin and yang, opening the door for effective Chinese medicine approaches without the adverse side effects that many Western sedative drugs produce (such as grogginess, motor impairment, or loss of mental clarity) and no risk of dependence. Furthermore, one-size-fits-all sedative drugs lack long-term effectiveness and fail to address the

underlying condition, often resulting in less than optimal results compared to the traditional Chinese medicine approach of alleviating sleep issues based on specific underlying causes.

Although the basic concept is quite simple, pattern differentiation allows for a more nuanced and personalized intervention. Though the dynamic always includes the Heart's ability to "store the spirit," Chinese medicine categorizes several different patterns that inhibit our goal of achieving rest. Examples include:

• Feelings of heat and pressure in the chest, causing difficulty falling asleep

• Anxiety and restlessness that can prevent sleep or cause frequent waking

• An inability to return to sleep

Digestive problems can even be linked to sleep disruption, which is why certain formulas may focus on the digestive function while also benefiting insomnia.

Sometimes, patterns of sleep disruption are rooted in early life, especially adverse childhood experiences. These individuals may be prone to fear overtaking the sleep process, intrusive thoughts entering the mind or preventing a return to sleep, or nightmares that disrupt sleep. This represents a fundamental disruption of the Kidney and Heart: The light of awareness is overtaken by dark tides of fear, with every sleep event a foray into the unknown.

Sleep is, paradoxically, one of the most important activities of our lives and is a cornerstone of health and wellness. Rather than simply trying to sedate the body, Chinese medicine seeks to create a harmonious environment internally, in the same manner that we recognize how important a safe and relaxing external environment can be for sleep. With Chinese medicine, we become empowered to establish that peace within, whether with herbal medicine, acupuncture, acupressure, footbaths, or mind-body practices.

Early Bedtime and the Body Clock

The most essential pillar of health in traditional Chinese medicine is the importance of following your biological rhythm, including circadian (daily) rhythm, lunar rhythm, and seasonal rhythm. Over millennia, physicians throughout ancient China developed many theories to better understand these phenomena, as well as guidelines for putting them into practice. Among these guidelines, the most crucial is the traditional Chinese medicine body clock, a time chart that dedicates two-hour slots to the various Organ systems, during which blood circulation to that Organ peaks. This allows us to determine the most optimal time for sleep so that we will feel the most well rested.

One of the main takeaways from the body clock is that optimal bedtime should be between 9 and 11 p.m., as this is the time of San Jiao, or the "triple burner," representing the metabolic and endocrine systems, and that we should be fully asleep between 11 p.m. and 1 a.m., which is the time of the Gallbladder meridian, which represents our yang qi, essentially our energy. Chinese medicine's most emphasized key to health is adopting a bedtime no later than 11 p.m., which ensures we have adequate energy for the next day. Being asleep during the hours of 11 p.m. to 3 a.m. is considered critical to one's health and well-being; chronically staying up late is

considered damaging to both physical and mental health, and extremely taxing to liver function, in particular.

To skeptical night owls, the body clock's categorization of Organs into time slots may seem one of the most abstract and arbitrary rules of Chinese medicine. Surely, length of sleep matters more than the time one falls asleep? However, in recent years, modern scientific studies have demonstrated that there is, indeed, evidence to back these theories from ancient China. Not only is your sleep quality affected when you choose a sleep period contrary to the natural day-night rhythm, but your body also feels the effect—at the Organ level as well as the cellular level.

Take the heart, which, according to the TCM body clock, rules from 11 a.m. to 1 p.m. A 2016 research article indicates that blood pressure and heart rate reach their peaks during this period, as does the incidence of myocardial infarction, arrhythmia, angina pectoris, and sudden cardiac death. The researchers further explain that "cardiac burden rises to the highest point, and risks of exhausted heart [are] the highest with the highest incidence of morbidity" during this time period, indicating just how well the body clock theory understands our body's functions and optimal sleep time.

Recent studies also show that circadian rhythm disruption may induce or accelerate the onset of multiple diseases, including Alzheimer's, obesity, and diabetes, and is a risk factor for breast cancer. A new study from Washington University indicates that people showing evidence of preclinical Alzheimer's disease—more amyloid buildup in their brains—had more fragmentation in their

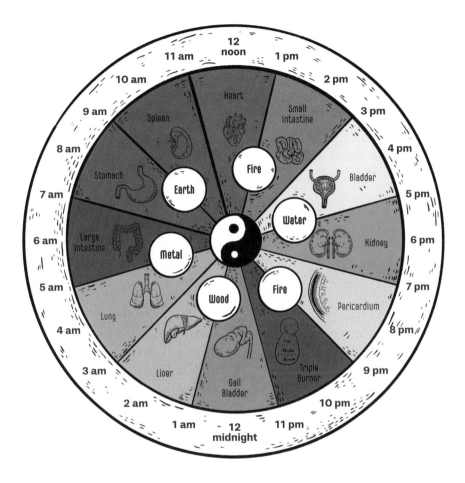

circadian activity patterns: more inactivity during the day and more activity at night. Although researchers have a long way to go before developing a full understanding of dementia, we know that Alzheimer's damage can take root in the brain fifteen to twenty years before symptoms appear. Low-quality sleep has also been found to promote inflammation and atherosclerosis, limiting blood flow not only to the heart but to all vital organs of the body. Lastly, multiple studies have demonstrated that centenarians tend to go to sleep early, further suggesting that a healthy sleep cycle can improve health and longevity.

If sleep is something you struggle with consistently, you might want to integrate traditional Chinese medicine wisdom into your routine and try these natural, time-tested solutions for insomnia.

Causes of Insomnia: Chinese Medicine Patterns

Insomnia in Chinese medicine is typically described in terms of patterns of heat, Blood Deficiency, and Yin Deficiency. One of the most commonly diagnosed causes of insomnia in Chinese medicine is referred to as Agitation of the Heart. This is primarily a heat pattern, where heat is understood to be any form of overwork of a bodily system, or an inflammatory process. This pattern can evolve from a feverish condition, like the common cold, that has caused thirst and a feeling of dryness, and perhaps left some inflammation behind in the chest after upper respiratory congestion. However, it is not limited to this. Cold, after all, is anything that inhibits the basic warming processes that defines health and vitality. So even harsh words that one cannot release and let go of can cause anguish in the Heart and inability to sleep, just like physical inflammation. But the overall sense would be one of dryness and pressure in the chest inhibiting relaxation.

Similarly, perhaps the most common form of insomnia has a unique term applied to it: Deficient Vexation. This refers to a condition where an internal source is the primary cause, and the inability to settle the mind, relax, and calm the nervous system is impaired over a longer period of time by overthinking, worry, mental or physical overwork, or preoccupation with an unresolved issue. All of that work is exhausting for the body and uses so many resources that the system becomes brittle and overly sensitive, as if the soothing functions of the body have become exhausted. Any kind of intense overstimulation can produce this, but when caused by worry or anxiety, there is often an even more

direct effect. The Liver is also implicated in this scenario, because Liver Blood is a term to describe the ability of the body to adapt and restore itself—a description of the literal circulatory effects regulating sleep, resulting in Liver Blood Deficiency.

Another pattern of intense insomnia is described as the "inability to lie down." This is a euphemism for a severe state of sleeplessness. This can also be described as the failure of the Heart and Kidney to communicate. In that case, the activity of the Heart-Mind cannot be quieted, and this would imply more pressing mental concerns. When Fire is raging, as if without restraining forces, it will be characterized by a kind of pressure and intensity that is more severe. Sadly, this type of intense disruption can even stem from early childhood, implying a long-term pattern of lifelong insomnia. It is often characterized by both an inability to initiate sleep due to profuse or intrusive thoughts, sometimes further worsened by easy waking and an inability to get back to sleep, and an inability to stay asleep. A telltale sign is dark circles under the eyes and a "wired" state. Sleep deprivation can be disastrous for health.

Thankfully, not all insomnia is this severe—day-to-day circumstances can also disrupt sleep. When simple stress is the culprit, the Liver's qi is often said to be stagnant. One way to describe this is as an irresistible force meeting an immovable object. Things like bills, work stress, interpersonal difficulties, perfectionism, or deadlines are all examples of stressors that can make falling asleep a challenge. When this happens, there might also be some digestive disturbances like loose stools, slight abdominal pain, or a stitch under the ribs. Sometimes that also follows late-night meals, convenience foods, or less healthy food choices, and this can lead to a related pattern where the difficulty of digesting—or even belching and reflux—can disrupt sleep. In that case, a pattern called Food Stagnation applies, and there is a long history of effective herbal formulas and even abdominal massages that can help alleviate this quickly.

Remedies for Insomnia

Herbal Formulas for Insomnia

It is important to note that Chinese herbal medicine for insomnia does not work like Western sleep drugs do—although some may contain sedative herbs, they do not focus only on sedating but on restoring your health and natural circadian rhythm. Therefore, you may not notice a difference the same night you start taking them, but you should start to see results within a few days of consistent use. Furthermore, dosages are usually split several times throughout the day—there is no need to worry about any drowsiness when taken earlier in the day because these do not function like sedatives. It is important to take the dosage as recommended by the formula manufacturer or licensed practitioner. The course of treatment may vary, but the goal is to restore your body's balance so that herbal medicine is no longer necessary. Take the formula for at least four weeks, then you may reduce your dosage or take only as needed. These formulas are also safe for long-term use.

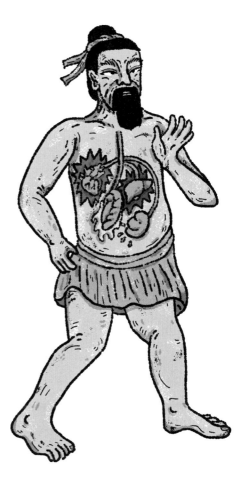

Conceptual illustration of different patterns in a body that contribute to insomnia

Suan Zao Ren Tang 酸枣仁汤 (Sour Jujube Seed Decoction)

Suan Zao Ren Tang is the most well-known and widely used sleep remedy in the Chinese canon. First appearing in the third-century text *Essential Prescriptions of the Golden Cabinet*, the formula treats a pattern of deficient vexation and the inability to sleep; in other words, when you feel fatigued and tired but are unable to fall asleep due to a restless mind and anxiety. A 2015 randomized, parallel-control trial found Suan Zao Ren Tang, combined with Zhi Zi Chi Tang (see page 60), to be more effective at reducing insomnia severity than benzodiazepines (lorazepam, Ativan). This formula also uniquely addresses dream-disturbed sleep, which can mean having profuse dreaming or even nightmares. There should be at least 48 grams per dose of Suan Zao Ren, or Sour Jujube Seed.

Herb	Function	Indications
Suan Zao Ren	Strengthens Liver Blood, calms spirit (shen)	Inability to sleep, excessive dreaming
Fu Ling	Calms spirit	Fright, palpitations
Gan Cao	Tonifies qi and yin, harmonizes	Grounding and centering
Zhi Mu	Nourishes Kidney, clears deficient heat, calms Heart	Tension, heat, nervous system inflammation
Chuan Xiong	Circulates Blood, alleviates depression	Stuck feelings, fixed ideas

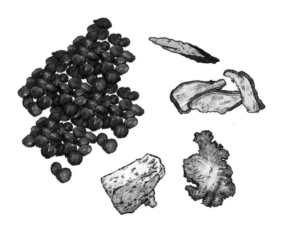

Jia Wei Xiao Yao San 加味消遥散 (Free and Easy Wanderer Plus)

Jia Wei means "added flavors" and refers to the addition of Zhi Zi and Mu Dan Pi to the very important formula Xiao Yao San—perhaps the most famous Liver Qi Stagnation formula used to treat any symptom that is made worse by stress, and certainly the most clinically researched. While many studies on this formula examine its effects on anxiety, a 2009 randomized, controlled study found that Jia Wei Xiao Yao provided benefits to subjective sleep quality comparable to a benzodiazepine. One hallmark of a Liver issue is that it is caused by stress, or the aftermath of stress—any time an immovable force meets an immovable object, stagnation is the result. Pain when pressing the ribs is a telltale sign. Over time, this can give rise to increased pressure and heat. Heat rises, and then affects the Heart, causing insomnia to accompany the irritability associated with the Liver.

Herb	Function	Indications
Chai Hu	Moves Wood, qi	Irritability, stress
Bai Shao	Eases tension, strengthens Blood	Muscle tension, emotional tension
Dang Gui	Tonifies Blood	Depression, menstrual irregularity
Bai Zhu	Tonifies Spleen	Loose stools
Fu Ling	Tonifies Spleen, transforms fluids	Fatigue
Bo He	Moves Liver Qi, cools	Emotional constraint
Sheng Jiang	Warms and dries Earth	Loose stools
Zhi Gan Cao	Harmonizes	Feelings of urgency and tension
Zhi Zi	Clears heat	Irritability, vexation
Mu Dan Pi	Cools Blood	Hot temper

Huang Lian E Jiao Tang 黃蓮阿膠湯 (Coptis and E Jiao Decoction)

Huang Lian E Jiao Tang is a critical formula for insomnia and is associated with Kidney Yin Deficiency. It supports blood and fluids, and descends Fire from the Heart back into the depth of stillness, where it is embraced by the deeply nourishing resources of egg yolks and beef gelatin. In the Qin and Han dynasties, beef gelatin was used to make E Jiao, which is recommended over other forms of E Jiao. This is suitable for chronic, enervating states of insomnia with symptoms such as inability to get to sleep due to racing thoughts and intense patterns of insomnia that can last all night, often with a long chronic history. As most formulas do not contain egg yolk, two large egg yolks will need to be added after—simply stir the raw egg yolks into the strained decoction when the temperature decreases. This formula may not be widely available.

Herb	Function	Indications
Huang Lian	Bitter taste descends Fire harassing the spirit (shen)	Insomnia, agitation, inability to rest
Huang Qin	Courses Fire so it moves freely and promotes metabolism	Irritability, restlessness
E Jiao (gelatin)	Deeply nourishes yin and Blood	Taxation, easily triggered, agitated
Bai Shao	Softens and eases tension	Muscle tension and stagnation
Ji Zi Huang (egg yolk)	Nourishes life force to restore nervous system	Lacking groundedness and internal resources

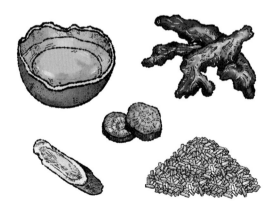

Tian Wang Bu Xin Dan 天王補心丹 **(Heavenly King Tonify the Heart Special Pills)**

Tian Wang Bu Xin Dan is a complex formula used to treat anxiety and insomnia. Originally formulated as honey pills, it is still widely available in this form. The formula is deeply nourishing to fluids and Blood (yin substances), clears deficient heat brought about by mental exhaustion and overwork, and calms the spirit (shen) to treat restlessness and insomnia. Mental symptoms would also be accompanied by dryness and feelings of heat. If you experience frequent waking throughout the night (key to this formula) and racing thoughts, as well as anxiety during the day, try this remedy.

Herb	Function	Indications
Sheng Di Huang Tian Men Dong Mai Men Dong Xuan Shen	Nourishes yin fluids, nutritive	Restlessness, dry throat and mouth, night sweats
Wu Wei Zi	Calms spirit (shen)	Overthinking
Bai Zi Ren	Calms spirit, nourishes Heart Blood	Poor memory, difficulty concentrating
Suan Zao Ren	Calms spirit, nourishes Liver Blood	Excessive dreaming, wandering thoughts
Dang Gui	Moves and nourishes Blood	Pallor, dryness, brittle nails
Long Yan Rou	Nourishes Liver Blood	Poor memory, difficulty focusing
Dan Shen	Strengthens Heart qi and Blood	Palpitations, insomnia
Fu Ling	Strengthens Spleen, calms spirit	Insomnia palpitations due to phlegm, or water metabolism
Yuan Zhi	Connects Heart and Kidney	Restlessness, palpitations with anxiety, disorientation
Jie Geng	Opens chest, circulates qi	Chest congestion
Zhu Sha	Sedates and calms spirit	Restlessness, irritability

Zhi Zi Chi Tang 梔子豉湯 (Gardenia and Fermented Soybean Decoction)

Zhi Zi Chi Tang is a uniquely simple remedy comprising two herbs: Zhi Zi (Gardenia Fruit) and Dan Dou Chi (Fermented Soybeans), which is a common food. Combined, the two medicinals reduce irritability and feelings of heat in the chest that could prevent you from settling down to sleep. If you are experiencing an overworked mind, a feeling of heat and constraint, or a lot of tossing and turning, you will likely benefit from the relatively gentle releasing action of the formula.

Herb	Function	Indications
Zhi Zi	Reduces irritability, cools Blood	Irritability, constraint
Dan Dou Chi	Clears heat	Vexation, insomnia

Gan Cao Xie Xin Tang 甘草瀉心湯 (Licorice Decoction to Drain the Epigastrium)

Gan Cao Xie Xin Tang is a representative formula that addresses the role of the digestive system in sleep disturbance. Combinations of cold and hot stimuli in the stomach can give rise to a painful epigastric sensation. This disruption of the ascending and descending functions of digestion can exhibit heat and dryness above the diaphragm that affects the Heart, causing vexation and insomnia, along with loose stools and gurgling derived from cold and deficiency below.

Herb	Function	Indications
Zhi Gan Cao	Tonifies qi, harmonizes	Vexation, insomnia
Ban Xia	Dries damp, resolves phlegm	Nausea, epigastric pain
Huang Qin	Moves and redirects heat	Inflammation
Huang Lian	Sedates Fire in Stomach and Heart	Insomnia
Ren Shen	Generates qi and fluids	Dryness
Da Zao	Warms Earth with sweet taste	Bloating, poor appetite
Gan Jiang	Warms Earth, dispels damp	Loose stools, gurgling, bloating

Acupressure for Insomnia

When it comes to using acupressure for insomnia, we focus on points that are known to calm the mind, relax the body, and promote overall relaxation. Simply press on these points or massage them using your hands, a gua sha tool, or an acupressure stick, pressing for about two minutes until you feel relaxed and calm.

Anmian

Anmian, which means "peaceful sleep," is one of the most significant extra points for insomnia. It is found behind the ear, below the bony mastoid process, in a small depression. Circular pressure here will ease tension and can also alleviate tension in the neck and shoulders that inhibits relaxation.

Taixi

Taixi is the source point of the Kidney, which means it has a direct effect on the Organ. As such, it governs consolidation and groundedness. The point is midway between the Achilles tendon and the height of the ankle bone. Firm pressure and concentrated attention to the breath can be deeply nourishing and calming. Visualizing the breath traveling to the heel, according to the saying that the sage breathes from the heels, can help the spirit (shen) settle and ease into restful sleep.

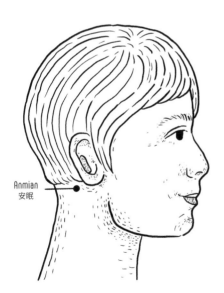

Anmian
安眠

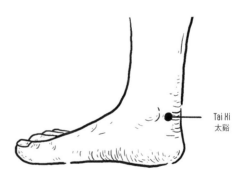

Tai Xi
太谿

Sanyinjiao

Sanyinjiao is found one hand's width above the ankle bone, in the inside of the lower leg. There is a depression there that is often sensitive to pressure. This point is strongly indicated for any menstrual pain, and it can also ease tension and calm an overactive, worried, irritable, or even fearful state that inhibits sleep. As the meeting of three yin channels, the emotions attributed to the Spleen, Liver, and Kidney can all benefit from firm, pulsing pressure here.

Yintang

Yintang is an extra point found above and between the eyebrows. It is one of the most relaxing points, promoting a sense of calm and quieting an overactive mind. Stroking downward will also help direct the qi downward and induce a state of ease.

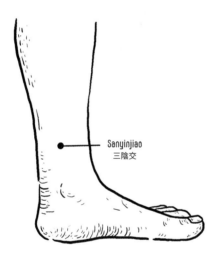

Sanyinjiao
三陰交

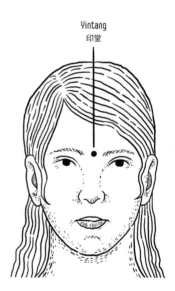

Yintang
印堂

Foot Soaks for Insomnia

A unique aspect of Chinese culture is the emphasis on everyday wellness. While in the West, footbaths may be an occasional indulgence, this is a daily routine for a large part of the Chinese population to improve sleep and boost immunity.

All across the Chinese-speaking world, there are foot massage establishments, popular from morning to late night and available at every price range. One thing all foot massage spots have in common is that they always start the process with a hot footbath. Even Sun Simiao (孙思邈), known as the King of Medicine, recommended "warm feet to help calm the heart so people could fall asleep" in his seventh-century text, *Essentials Formulas Worth a Thousand Gold Pieces*.

This often begs the question from Westerners about why footbaths, in particular, are the preferred nighttime wellness ritual—shouldn't full-body baths be just as good for our health, if not better? The answer is a resounding no. Long full-body baths are best avoided according to traditional Chinese medicine because they cause excess heating and sweating, which is overly draining on the body. Hot footbaths, on the other hand, help the entire body relax, thanks to the seventy-plus acupressure points on the feet, and effectively lower core body temperature without causing increased sweating. Numerous research studies also support the idea that hot footbaths are effective for improving both sleep quality and duration. One study on menopausal women with poor sleep summarized footbaths as a "safe, simple, and nonpharmacological method to improve sleep quality." *Footbaths are safe for the majority of people, but diabetics should avoid them.*

Those in the know also regularly incorporate herbs into their footbath (in the form of herbal sachets) for even greater health benefits, often including the anti-inflammatory herb mugwort or the pain-relieving, circulation-promoting ginger.

Note: You can get inexpensive soaking basins for footbaths at most Asian grocery stores, online, or, in a pinch, you can even use an insulated food delivery bag, which is similar to a foldable footbath basin.

To get the best benefits from your foot soak, follow these instructions:

1. Shortly before bedtime, fill a basin with hot (104°F to 110°F, or 40°C to 43°C) water to completely cover your ankles. The temperature should be very hot but not scalding. Use a thermometer if you have difficulty gauging temperature. Add an herbal sachet to the bath, if you like. Have a towel nearby.

2. Submerge your feet in the water and soak for 15 to 30 minutes. One thermoregulatory analysis found that the optimal duration of a footbath at 107.6°F, or 42°C, was 24 minutes, when sweating just occurs.

3. If the water turns cold, boil some water in a kettle and slowly add it to your footbath until it becomes hot again.

4. With a towel, dry your feet immediately at the end of your footbath.

5. Hydrate afterward by drinking some warm or room-temperature water.

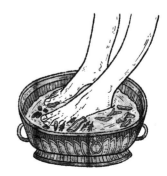

Tui Na 推拿

Tui na (or tuina), one of the oldest forms of bodywork and a well-known modality of Chinese medicine, focuses on removing blockages leading to pain and illness through a combination of massage, physical therapy, and chiropractic techniques in the Western lexicon. A tui na session may include acupressure, myofascial release, stretching, compression, and more and can involve hands, arms, elbows, and sometimes even knees and feet—in some establishments, you'll see parallel bars installed high over the massage table for practitioners to hold on to while they "step" on your back. Although this book emphasizes healing modalities you can do yourself, tui na warrants a special mention because it can be extremely effective for insomnia. (However, there are also a variety of self-massage tools easily available online, as well as electric neck–upper back massagers that can reduce tension in a pinch.)

A 2018 meta-analysis of eleven studies determined that tui na can produce more significant efficacy in treating primary insomnia compared with other traditional Chinese medicine therapies and oral administration of Western medication, especially the combination of head and back tui na. Similarly, a 2023 meta-analysis of eighteen studies determined that tui na can significantly improve the sleep quality of patients with primary insomnia, and it was more effective than other treatments, including benzodiazepines, acupuncture, gua sha scraping, auricular acupressure, and Suan Zao Ren Decoction.

The treatments are usually no-frills and, so, relatively inexpensive compared to spa massages. If you suffer from insomnia, ask your masseuse to focus on the back and head and skip the legs. Book full-body massages an hour or more after eating, and remember to hydrate well afterward with warm water.

Five Element Music Therapy for Insomnia

While Five Element music therapy is still considered a relatively new therapy—and one nearly unheard of in the West—through a number of studies over the years, we know that insomnia is one of the conditions it is most effective in treating. Following, I have modified the expert-tailored protocol designed by a team of researchers at Shanghai University of Traditional Chinese Medicine and Shanghai Jiao Tong University School of Medicine for a study that evaluated anxiety and quality of sleep of asymptomatic COVID patients in quarantine. The protocol was designed with five different songs to be played at five times throughout the day, carefully chosen to enhance the functions of the five Organ systems. Participants were instructed to rest in a supine (lying face-up) position with eyes lightly closed while listening to the music—however, you can also take in the music therapy while sitting down.

Study participants also performed Baduanjin qigong exercises daily. The researchers reported that they were satisfied with the patients' changes in emotions and sleep quality after about seven days.

Here is the Shanghai medical research team's protocol, with additional musical tracks I have added that correspond to the specified tone/functions prescribed at the various times.

1. **First thing in the morning:** Play Yu-tone music for 30 minutes:

   "Plum-Blossom in Three Movements"
   "Zhaojun's Resentment"
   "Song of the Past"

2. **Afternoon:** Play Shang-tone music for 30 minutes:

   "White Snow in Early Spring"
   "A Parting Tune with a Thrice Repeat Refrain"
   "A Moonlit Night on the Spring River"
   "Yangguan Sandie"

3. **Post-dinner in the evening:** Play music with Wood quality for 30 minutes:

   "A Song on the Frontier Fortress"
   "Evening Song in the Fishing Boat" also translated as "Fisherman's Song at Dusk"

4. **Before bed:** Play Zhi-tone music for 30 minutes:

   "Daughter's Love"
   "Autumn Moon in the Han Palace"
   "Su Wu Tending the Sheep"
   "Butterfly"

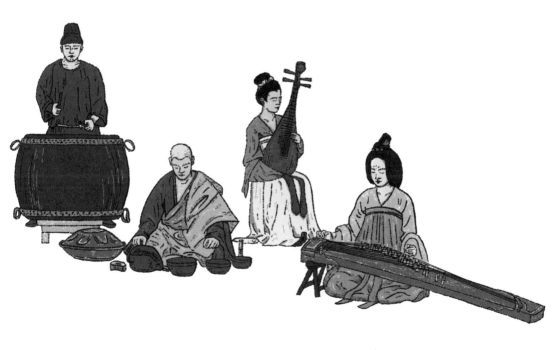

Qigong Exercises for Insomnia

As you've learned, from a Chinese medical perspective, insomnia can originate from a variety of factors. Rather than address all of the potential causes in one set of exercises, the qigong regimen here is presented as a valuable adjunct therapy designed to calm the mind to prepare it for sleep. Repeated frequently, the series will calm and settle the mind.

All exercises can be performed either standing, seated in a chair, or lying down in a supine position. If at any stage during the exercise you become sleepy, as the mind and body begins to relax, cease the exercise, close your eyes, and go to sleep. *These exercises are best performed sequentially*, but can also be performed individually if one or multiple exercises cannot be performed for any reason.

Leg and Foot Massage

1. Self-massage the legs, downward, focusing on releasing any areas of tightness.

2. Massage the ankles and soles of the feet with the intention of leading your qi to the area.

3. Stop the massage when a gentle warmth is felt in both feet.

Healing Xu Sound

1. With both hands over the qihai point (about 3 inches, or 7.5 cm, under the navel) or by the sides of the body, inhale deeply.

2. Upon exhaling, make the sound "Xu" (pronounced *shuuuuuu*, very slowly

and gently, releasing air from between the teeth so the sound lasts as long as possible. It should both sound and feel like air being released from a hole in a tire. With each exhale, focus on a descending motion happening in the body, starting at the face, moving down the torso, legs, and down into the feet.

3. Repeat 9 to 108 times.

Yongquan 涌泉 Point Respiration

1. Focus on the Yongquan point (located in the depression found in the top one-third of the sole of the foot between the second and third metatarsal joints. It can be easily located as a depression formed when the toes are pulled toward the sole of the foot, and is about one-third of the way down from the top of the toes to the bottom of the heel) on the soles of the feet.

2. Breathing with long, slow, deep breaths, try to sense the point expanding on your inhale and contracting on the exhale.

3. Repeat until you feel tired enough to sleep.

Intentional Relaxation Sequence

With the eyes half closed or fully closed, focus the mind on various parts of the body, in this order, and relax the muscles, ligaments, and joints. Any point where you find it difficult to focus your attention is likely a place of significant blockage and can be focused on for longer. If you find you can't put your mind in a certain area at all, combine this mental practice with gentle self-massage in the area.

1. Focus on the wrists, palms, hands, and fingers. Relax these areas for a minimum of 9 long, slow, deep breaths, releasing any tension. Over time, with repeated practice, you should be able to feel the area expand gently with your inhale and contract with the exhale.

2. Repeat this process with the feet, ankles, and soles of the feet.

3. Move to the shoulders, releasing tension around the scapula, pectoral muscles, collarbones, trapezius muscle, and shoulder joint capsule.

4. Move to the elbows, releasing tension at the font, back, and either side of the joint.

5. Focus on the hips and buttocks, relaxing the muscles around this area.

6. Move your attention to the perineum, and repeat the same process here.

7. Relax the muscles around and down the cervical spine, starting from the base at the back of the skull and slowly releasing any tension downward until you reach the first thoracic joint.

8. Bring your attention to the top of the sternum at the base of the throat and release tension there down the center of the body, down through the sternum, the xiphoid process, and through the centerline of the abdomen, down through the navel, and stopping at qihai, about 3 inches (7.5 cm) under the navel.

9. Move your attention to the Zhongwan acupuncture point, located in this same centerline about halfway between the navel and the xiphoid process, and repeat the relaxation process.

10. Move to the knees, and release tension from the front, back, and both sides of the joints.

11. Move your attention back to the occiput of the skull, and work your way down the muscles and ligaments of the entire spine, down to the sacrum, continuing to release the muscles of the perineum from back to front, and up through the genitals, stopping again at the qihai point. Breathe slowly and quietly with your focus in this area for a minimum of 18 long, slow, deep breaths.

Conclusion

Since these chapters are organized by Western terminology, if you are suffering from insomnia, you may also want to explore chapter 5, Depression, chapter 6, Anxiety, and chapter 9, Trauma, which may overlap with insomnia.

In the next chapter, we will explore TCM healing modalities for depression.

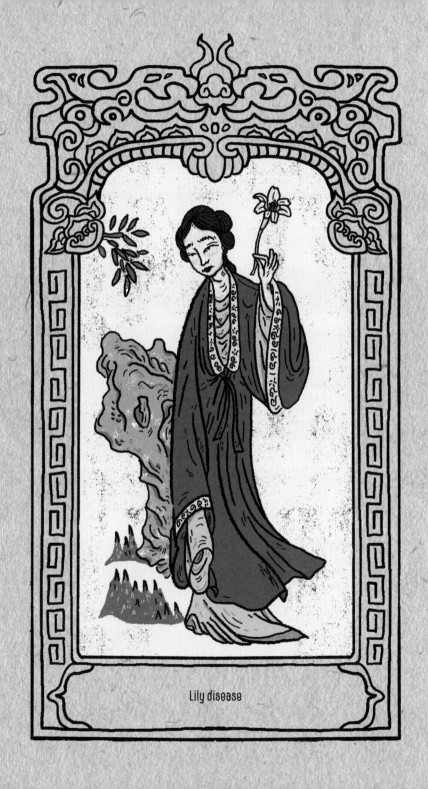

Lily disease

CHAPTER 5

DEPRESSION

Depression can feel hopeless and isolating, especially when you consider mounting new evidence that the standardized treatment—selective serotonin reuptake inhibitor (SSRIs)—work no better than placebo for 85 percent of people. Those suffering from depression may be pleasantly surprised to learn that this is one of the most time-tested and widely studied areas within Chinese herbal medicine, with some herbal formulas even outperforming Western prescription medications for depression in double-blind, placebo-controlled trials. In fact, the most popular formula in all of Chinese medicine is one that is most frequently prescribed for mood disorders, including depression and anxiety, and studies have found that its effects are felt sooner than SSRIs, with further systematic review concluding there were no adverse effects. Furthermore, some of the earliest case studies from Chinese medicine were for depression, with one that dates back to 160 BCE.

An Historian's Overview of Depression in Traditional Chinese Medicine

In ancient China, according to the text *Shuowen jiezi xizhuan*, the character 人—meaning "person"—was interpreted as "the concentrated and refined lively material upon the separation of heaven and Earth." The common belief was that people attained longevity by living in harmony with nature, accommodating their cravings and desires within the natural environment, and that only then would they remain free from sorrow or anger. Conversely, if the energy, or qi, within the body or between the body and the environment is imbalanced, feelings of depression may arise.

"Depression," as a medical term, is a relatively modern one that is typically characterized by persistent sadness, hopelessness, difficulty concentrating, exhaustion, and alterations in food consumption and sleep patterns. However, various forms of depression have had a long history in traditional Chinese medical texts, with case studies and records showing they were often successfully treated using well-known Chinese medicinal remedies. One of the earliest mentions of depression can be found in Sima Qian's monumental text *Records of the Grand Historian*, written between the late second and early first century BCE, which documented a disorder called "Qi Block" (or Qi Stagnation) that resulted from depression and an aggrieved Heart, and was treated with an herbal formula whose action was to move qi.

Around the first century BCE, the *Inner Classic of the Yellow Emperor* already recommended acupuncture as a remedy for depression and explained how to balance the Five Emotions (joy, anger, sadness, anxiety, and fear), which became the cornerstone of Chinese psychology. Zhang Zhongjing's *Shanghanlun* recorded two types of depression known as Lily Disease and Visceral Agitation, with respective cures: the decoction featuring the herb lily bulb (see page 74), and the decoction of licorice, wheat, and jujube (see page 77). These remedies are still widely employed by Chinese medicine physicians in treating depression today.

In the seventh century, Daoist physician Sun Simiao considered Wind (movement of the qi in nature or within the body) as something having a detrimental effect on the Spirit-Mind. Since Wind tends to invade the head—the uppermost part of the body—signs of having an "evil wind" include persistent feelings of anxiety or emptiness, body pain, eating disorder, fear, headache, insomnia, irritability, restlessness, and sadness. Sun Simiao provided a series of Life Prolonging Decoctions to dispel the "evil wind" and regain a clear head.

Since the eleventh century and continuing to today, Qi Stagnation (decrease in the normal activity of qi) came to be seen as the primary factor causing depression. The famous fourteenth-century physician Zhu Danxi believed that Qi Stagnation was the origin of all disease. Aside from herbal medicine and acupuncture, Zhu Danxi was notable for being one of the first physicians to offer psychotherapy talking sessions in his clinical practice as a treatment for depression.

From the seventeenth century onward, depression was most commonly linked to Liver Qi Stagnation or "constraint" (with Liver referring to a metaphorical part of a traditional Chinese medical visceral system, not the actual bodily organ), believed to be caused by strains such as anger and frustration, as well as unfulfilled desires. It was most commonly treated with Si Ni San (Four Reversals Powder, page 74) or Xiao Yao San (Free and Easy Wanderer Powder, page 75) or its modified formula, Jia Wei Xiao Yao San (see page 75), to rectify Liver Qi and resolve depression. The latter of these formulas remains the most popular one today, especially in wan (pill) form. Using these ancient, time-tested remedies, we can heal the depressed Liver and achieve harmony within our body and with the world around us.

A Clinician's Approach to Depression in Traditional Chinese Medicine

When it comes to depression, the most common cause of low mood and other symptoms is stagnation, Yu (郁 / 鬱). The image portrayed in the traditional form of this character (right) is a thicket, like thorny wild blackberries. Another way to describe this is an irrepressible force meeting an immovable object. Whenever you feel like you are stuck and don't see a way out, you experience stagnation. In contrast to anxiety, which can feel like a rush of uncontrolled energy, depression is a sign that the energy has been exhausted, or is unable to move. Both the Lung and the Liver are implicated in promoting a feeling of ease and freedom in the body, through the regularity of breath and physical feelings of flow and suppleness. Let's take a closer look at both in relation to depression.

The Lung

In the earliest Chinese medical texts, depression was attributed to the Lung—especially because this Organ system is associated with grief, and grief prolonged becomes melancholy and depression. Sighing and yawning are physical responses that illustrate how the body tries to release held emotions or exhaustion. The connection between physical response and emotion may have led to the conclusion that the Lung is involved, because both of these responses are essentially exaggerations of the breath.

The Liver

Over time, the relationship between free and easy movement—or its opposite—was attributed to the Liver. There are a number of classical medical references to the Liver as the source of dynamic movement and free-flowing energy: The Liver is likened to a general who is able to strategize and seize the moment. In depression, it can seem impossible to see a favorable outcome for yourself, and even more difficult to take action. This has an effect on blood circulation and disrupts patterns of rest and activity. You might feel tired but agitated, sleepy but unable to fall sleep, and lose interest in things you previously enjoyed or lack the energy to do them. Another term related to the Liver is knotted qi, which can often show up as pain in the body, especially through muscle tension in the neck and upper back and around the ribs. These are all aspects of depression.

If you can dream big dreams and envision great things but lack the physical energy to fulfill those plans, depression will result. Since the Liver is like a general, you might look at other people achieving their dreams and feel envious. Envy can turn into spite and negativity, both of which cause unpleasant physical feelings and create a feedback loop of suffering turned inward, further sapping energy. Sadly, the initial injury can come from emotional or physical abuse that over-

whelmed the nervous system, or even illnesses like Lyme disease or mononucleosis.

A commonly overlooked aspect of depression stems from Yang Deficiency. This means that instead of feeling as though you're at an impasse, you might just feel totally exhausted. But there is an even deeper aspect of this, too. Chinese medicine is unique in its understanding of the role that early life experiences can play in later life. For example, birth trauma, adverse childhood experiences, and dysfunctional family dynamics can all result in depression. All of these experiences share one thing in common with the previous types: You can feel stuck and powerless to change the past. It is common for people to suddenly realize that some past aspect of their life has produced negative consequences, which they feel unable to change, and then fall into a depression.

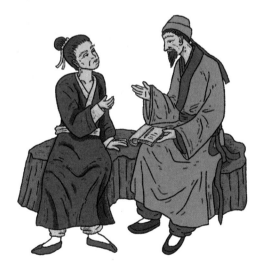

Talking cures, an early form of psychotherapy, in Ancient China

For example, you might feel that your needs were overlooked when you were a child. If so, you might be deeply invested in finding a partner to meet your needs and, in the absence of such a partner, become depressed. The loss of a caregiving partner is also a form of grief. This cycle could repeat until you discover through further introspection that the ultimate resources lie within you. But until that happens, there can be hopeless feelings and depressive episodes.

Fortunately, the supplementing, revitalizing herbs used in some herbal formulas for depression can help someone feel the internal warmth and energy to support that inner work and alleviate the physical pain and exhaustion accompanying depression. Different experiences influence particular Organ systems in the body, resulting in distinct patterns we can recognize, treat, and resolve. In the following section, look for the pattern that best describes your situation.

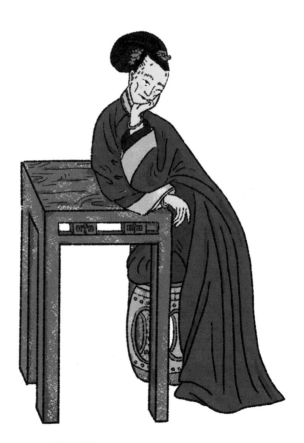

Ancient Chinese woman with Yang deficiency

Causes of Depression: Chinese Medicine Patterns

In traditional Chinese medicine, there are a number of patterns associated with depression, and identifying the pattern that encompasses your symptoms and experience is crucial to finding the right treatment. In the work of Dr. Leon Hammer, one of the pioneers of Chinese medicine psychology in the West, this is elaborated into several diagnostic patterns based on a subtle and sophisticated framework that identifies patterns of deficiency and excess for each phase. However, to make it easy to understand and relate to your experience, the following addresses a few of the most common patterns related to depression.

Liver Qi Stagnation

As previously mentioned, the Liver is strongly connected to feelings of stuckness and frustration that can be a part of depression. Liver Qi Stagnation is the most common diagnosis related to the term "Yu," discussed previously. You might have increased feelings of irritability and physical agitation that suggest heat has developed from the initial stagnation. Or, stress might affect your digestion, causing irregular bowel movements or bloating in addition to the stress response. Many of the corresponding formulas address symptoms of emotional lability (rapid changes in mood), unstable moods, and hopelessness.

Visceral Agitation

In addition to Liver patterns, the classical term "Visceral Agitation" explains feelings of overwhelm, sadness, and grief that are consistent with both depression and anxiety.

Blood Deficiency

Blood Deficiency, especially related to the Liver and its circulatory regulating function, shows itself as the feeling of cold hands and feet—clinicians understand this to mean any circumstance where pain and discomfort, a history of abuse, or an inability to connect to full self-expression is related to blood circulation and a feeling of warmth and vitality in the body.

Kidney Yang Deficiency

Kidney Yang Deficiency is, perhaps, the pattern most akin to major depression: If you want to sleep all the time and feel deep hopelessness and fatigue, then Kidney Yang Deficiency might be the Chinese medicine pattern that best fits your depression.

Remedies for Depression

Herbal Formulas for Depression

In the experience of clinicians, the following herbal formulas are acceptable to take even if you are currently on other medications, including SSRIs (as previously mentioned, space these out an hour in between). Refer to chapter 3, which provides more detail on how to take herbal formulas.

Si Ni San 四 逆 散 (Four Reversals Powder)

This ancient formula from the *Shanghanlun* is a marvelous example of sheer focus and power to move stagnation. A principal indication for this formula is cold hands and feet, with emotional depression, irritability, and feeling stuck. Cold hands and feet can seem like a unexpected symptom to associate with depression, but if your qi is not coursing enough to give free rein to bodily warmth, then it is a sure sign. Pain in the ribs and back are also telltale signs. The four herbs in this formula guarantee that, like the Taiji symbol, upward/outward vitality and inward/downward awareness will liberate your feelings of hopelessness.

Herb	Function	Indications
Chai Hu	Powerfully unblocks Liver and moves qi, ascending (or activating) movement (effect)	Distention and pain, irritability, negativity
Zhi Shi	Descending (or calming) movement and releases knotted qi	Pain in ribs and abdomen, constipation, tension
Bai Shao	Descending (or calming) movement and releases knotted qi	Muscle tension, hardened attitude, fixed ideas
Zhi Gan Cao	Harmonizes and strengthens Earth resources	Bitterness, lack of resiliency

Bai He Zhi Mu Tang 百合知母湯 (Lily Bulb Decoction)

This formula represents a group of formulas that treat a pattern called Lily Disease, or Bai He Bing (百合病). It involves a quality of internal discomfort, mental agitation, and mood swings, all centered on basic aspects of life: wanting to sleep but being unable to, wanting to eat but repulsed by everything, unable to regulate even your body temperature, and wanting to be active but feeling too agitated to do so. Those who suffer from these symptoms may benefit from this simple formula.

Herb	Function	Indications
Bai He	Nourishes Lung, Heart, and Pericardium, calms spirit (shen)	Dissatisfaction, emotional tension and lability, suffering that is hard to even identify
Zhi Mu	Nourishes and calms Kidney, clears heat and agitation	Restlessness, unhappiness

Xiao Yao San, or its modification, Jia Wei Xiao Yao San, 逍遙散 (Free and Easy Wanderer, Free and Easy Wanderer Plus)

This classic formula is the most researched and proven remedy for depression in the world. Its name refers to the wonderful effects the remedy has in supporting circulation as well as softer emotions (Blood), digestive function, and inner resources (Spleen Qi) while also stabilizing mood (Liver Qi Stagnation). A 2001 randomized, double-blind, placebo-controlled study found that for mild to moderate depression with anxiety, this formula was as effective as sertraline (Zoloft), but its effect was felt sooner and was deemed safer and less expensive than its Western medicine counterpart. Xiao Yao San and Jia Wei Xiao Yao San are also extremely safe—a systematic review across twenty-six randomized trials involving 1,837 patients showed no adverse effects. It is especially useful for premenstrual syndrome or depressed feelings occurring around menses, as well as fatigue, irritability, and irregular bowel movements, all of which are worse with stress. It is notably derived from the previously listed formula, Si Ni San.

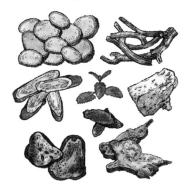

Herb	Function	Indications
Chai Hu	Frees the Liver, alleviates depression	Stress, pain, irritability
Bai Shao	Softens tension, promotes ease, nourishes Blood	Tension, spasm, rigidity
Dang Gui	Nourishes Blood and promotes circulation	Labile emotions, easily irritated, moderate pain, menstrual complaints
Bai Zhu	Benefits the Spleen, alleviates Dampness	Irregular bowel movements, abdominal bloating
Fu Ling	Percolates and strengthens	Irregular bowel movements, poor appetite
Bo He	Soothes Liver and opens qi movement	Stress, tension, easily triggered, agitation, hot temper
Sheng Jiang	Dries Dampness, warms digestion, settles stomach	Indigestion
Zhi Gan Cao	Harmonizes	Lack of centeredness

Dang Gui Si Ni Tang 當歸四逆湯 **(Dang Gui Decoction for Frigid Extremities)**

Although it is not commonly thought of as a depression formula, clinicians' experience identifies this is as unmatched in providing relief. The key symptoms that would indicate its use are a thin pulse and cold hands and feet. Together, these indicate that there is a subtle inhibition of blood circulation—not so much its volume and substance but in the force that drives it to warm and nourish the whole body. Negative self-talk is considered an aspect of depression, but this is often derived from the fixed ideas foisted on us when we attempt to express our selfhood; poor self-esteem often stems from external mistreatment and expectations forced upon us. This formula can awaken a driving strength toward self-expression, alleviate physical pain (such as in fibromyalgia), and promote circulation, helping you become so rooted and embodied that you can stand up to anything. *Avoid this formula if you have kidney disease.*

Herb	Function	Indications
Dang Gui	Promotes circulation, nourishes Liver Blood	Pain, cold hands and feet, diminished self-esteem
Xi Xin	Warms the channels, promotes microcirculation	Symptoms of withdrawal and guardedness, muscle pain
Mu Tong	Opens the vessels to promote circulation	Pain, cold hands and feet
Gui Zhi	Warms the body and promotes yang expression	Pain in the neck and back, tension, cold constriction, vulnerability to external stimuli
Bai Shao	Nourishes Blood, eases tension, develops resources	Tension, pain
Zhi Gan Cao	Harmonizes and nourishes the center	Lack of energy, fatigue
Da Zao	Tonifies qi and Blood	Difficulty concentrating, low focus, dry skin, pale skin

Gan Mai Da Zao Tang 甘麥大棗湯 (Licorice Wheat Jujube Decoction)

This two-thousand-year-old formula treats the pattern Visceral Agitation. The symptoms are very evocative: sorrow, weeping, acting as if possessed by spirits, yawning, and stretching. This is the most important formula for grief, the loss of a loved one, and breakups. When you feel like you cannot stop crying, this is the formula to reach for. These food-grade herbs act like a warm chicken soup for your spirit and will ease the discomfort of immovable emotion lodged in the body and mind that leaves you feeling overwhelmed. *Avoid this formula if you have celiac disease or gluten intolerance, as it contains wheat.*

Herb	Function	Indications
Fu Xiao Mai	Tonifies Heart and Liver, calms the mind	Visceral Agitation, unrest, aggravation, grief
Da Zao	Strengthens Blood	Heightened sensitivity, easily overwhelmed
Gan Cao	Tonifies qi	Lack of self-restraint, uncentered emotion

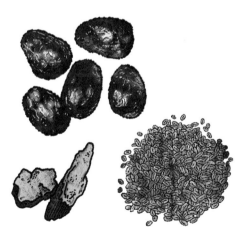

Zhen Wu Tang 真武湯 (True Warrior Decoction)

This formula, like Dang Gui Si Ni Tang (see page 76), is another that is not widely recognized for symptoms of depression. As its name suggests, it will help you find the energy to emerge from the darkness when immersed in the cold, watery depths of depression, or depression secondary to advanced illness that can require a potent impulse to the Kidney as much as a pain-relieving and spirit-calming impulse. The Kidney is involved whenever there is a long-term, chronic condition: Major depression is one such condition, as significant as the Heart disease this formula is known to treat. *Avoid this formula if you tend to run hot.*

Herb	Function	Indications
Fu Ling	Promotes water metabolism, calms spirit (shen), dispels fear	Dizziness, urinary difficulty, edema
Fu Zi	Warms, strengthens Kidney	Cold feelings, fatigue, sleepiness, diminished life force
Bai Shao	Nourishes Blood	Pain, tension
Bai Zhu	Tonifies Spleen, transforms Dampness	Abdominal pain, bloating, loose stool
Sheng Jiang	Radiates warmth, warms Earth	Cold, heavy feeling

Acupressure for Depression

The following is a combination of acupoints that can relieve frustrations, instill calmness, and boost mood. Use your fingers or an acupressure stick for best results.

Siguan 四关 (Four Gates)

This is similar to the herbal formula Si Ni San (see page 74). It helps promote relaxation and eases depression and difficult emotions due to its overall effect of regulating the directional movement of the qi. Any time you feel stuck or frustrated, get qi moving with acupressure at acupoint Hegu (LI 4) and Tai Chong (LV 3). Both of these points can be sensitive.

- To find LV 3, draw the index finger on top of the foot from the web between the first and second toes to a point of sensitivity between the bones.

- To find LI 4, locate the similar location between the thumb and index finger.

- Start by holding LI 4, pressing and rotating the thumb, kneading the muscle for a few minutes.

- Proceed to LV 3, and stroke outward toward the toes with firm pressure; visualize your frustration leaving your body and being embraced by Earth.

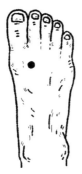

LV 3

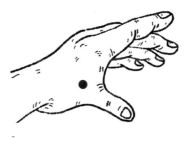

LI 4

Yintang 印堂 (Hall of Impression) and Tanzhong 膻中 (Chest Center)

This is another combination of points that can improve feelings of well-being and peace. Yintang is found between the eyebrows. Many people consider this the site of the third eye, and it can be helpful to think of it as calming and opening your eyes to new possibilities. Find Tanzhong (CV 17) in the center of the breastbone.

• With either hand, while pressing Yintang, feel a strong sense of peace as you focus your intention upon calming the spirit (shen).

• Continue pressing and visualize drawing those feelings of calm down into your chest.

• Now, with your dominant hand, press Tanzhong (CV 17) for a couple of minutes. Pay attention to your energetic state and what you are feeling, and do this until you feel better.

• Then, place both hands, palms down, on your chest and breathe in feelings of ease and liberation. Stay with the rise and fall of your chest, and let your attention become absorbed in relaxed peace.

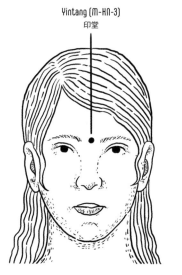

Yintang (M-HN-3)
印堂

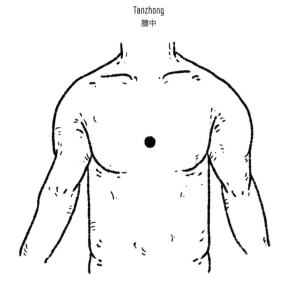

Tanzhong
膻中

Daoyin Exercises for Depression

Daoyin, a precursor to qigong, can be thought of as mind-body exercises that involve pulling or stretching your body. Chinese medicine has a rich history of medical treatises containing treatments and health protocols that Chinese medicine practitioners continue to read and follow today. One of these early works was the *Treatise on the Origins and Symptoms of Medical Disorders (Zhubing Yuanhou Lun)*, written by court physician Chao Yuanfang and his colleagues at the behest of the second Sui emperor in 610 CE. *Treatise* was significant in being the first medical text to attempt a comprehensive classification of diseases. It was also the first text to recommend therapeutic exercises, the majority of which were daoyin, as a treatment for specific disorders (as opposed to exercises meant for general health or longevity).

Following are several daoyin exercises recommended for depression, as translated from classical Chinese into English for the first time by medieval China historian Dolly Yang, PhD, author of an upcoming translation of *Zhubing Yuanhou Lun*. According to the text, "It is not suitable to move your qi after a big meal or when you are full of emotions such as joy, anger, sadness, or resentment. Practice moving your qi only at dawn when it is clear and quiet. It is the best way and will cure ten thousand diseases."

Exercise to Relieve Symptoms of Rising Qi
上氣候

This exercise can relieve congestion and compression of qi, which is associated with depression. It gets rid of qi in the Spine, Heart, and Lung—any congestion and compression will vanish and disperse.

Exercise to Relieve Symptoms of Knotted Qi
结气候

Knotted qi disorder is produced by worry and too much thinking. When the Heart is preoccupied, and the spirit (shen) has been seized, qi is stagnant and unmoving and becomes knotted inside. (This corresponds to the symptoms indicated under the Si Ni San formula.) To relieve knotted qi, which will also get rid of pain in both arms and in the back, follow these steps.

- Sit, lengthen your lumbus (lower back), and raise your left arm, palm facing up.

- Bring your right arm behind you, pressing your hand down.

- Inhale qi through your nose—do this as much as you can for 7 breaths (in and out).

- Between breaths, press your right hand down.

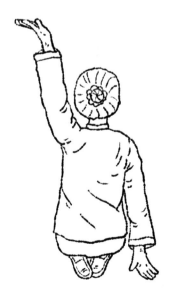

Symptoms of Liver Disorder

If you suffer from Liver disease (see previous clinical approach section on the Liver, page 71), you feel worried, sad, and unhappy. You may have anxious thoughts, or become annoyed and angry, or feel dizzy and have pain in your eyes.

Exhale qi while making a "he" sound; the symptoms will be cured. The sound "he" is pronounced as "her" without the r, not "he" as in the third person masculine pronoun.

- Bring both hands together behind your back. Press them against your lumbus (lower back), with fingers pointing up as much as possible.

- Shake and swing your arms and elbows backward and forward at least 7 times.

- Without changing your hand position, move your arms directly up and down, to and fro, as much as you can, twice 7 times (two sets of 7).

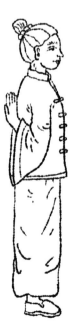

Tea for Depression

The consumption of tea for everyday health is well documented in classic Chinese texts, but newer studies have unearthed a connection to improved mood and lessening of depressive symptoms as well, making regular tea drinking a beneficial habit to support mental health. It's interesting to note that tea was initially introduced to the West as a medicinal with numerous curative effects. According to Thomas Garway, the first merchant to sell tea in England in 1657: "The Drink is declared to be most wholesome, preserving in perfect health untill extreme Old Age. It vanquisheth heavy Dreams, easeth the Brain, and strengtheneth the Memory."

Blue light emitted by phones and computers is associated with an increased risk of depression. In a fascinating new study, researchers noted that blue light exposure at night induced depression-like behaviors and gut microbiota disorders in a mouse model, and that pu'er tea intake significantly reshaped the gut microbiome (especially Bifidobacterium) and regulated the metabolism of short-chain fatty acids, which protect the integrity of the intestinal barrier. The authors of the study explained that the improvement in gut microbiome further reduced blood-brain barrier damage and alleviated neuroinflammation by inhibiting prototypical pro-inflammatory signaling pathways, which regulate neurotransmitters such as brain-derived neurotrophic factor and serotonin. By reshaping gut microbiota, reducing blood-brain barrier damage, and reducing neuroinflammation, pu'er tea can help alleviate symptoms of depression (read more about this in the Food Therapy section, starting on page 40). Because pu'er is a fermented tea, these new findings are not surprising given previous research indicating that microbes (such as Lactobacillus and Bifidobacteria species) associated with fermented foods may influence mental health.

For people who prefer other types of tea from the *Camellia sinensis* plant, such as oolong, green, black, or white tea, a 2015 meta-analysis of observational studies on tea drinking and depression found there was a linear association between tea consumption and the risk of depression, with an increment of three cups per day in tea consumption associated with a decrease in the risk of depression by 37 percent.

In another review of antidepressive effects of regular tea consumption, researchers thoroughly reviewed human trials, mouse models, and in vitro experiments. Their findings showed that the constituents found in all major tea types, predominantly L-theanine, polyphenols, and polyphenol metabolites, are capable of functioning through multiple pathways simultaneously to collectively reduce the risk of depression.

Good news for tea drinkers! You may also be interested to learn about tea's other effects in chapter 6, Anxiety.

Feng Shui for Depression

Feng shui, literally meaning "wind and water," is an ancient theory that holds that an individual's environment affects their internal state. Feng shui is based on the concept of qi, which, according to *Book of Burial*, functions like the flow of air representing the breath of nature and the energy of life. It should also be recognized that feng shui is not a superstition because it has a logical relationship between cause and effect.

While most people in the West have heard of feng shui, few seem to know its principles. Historically, feng shui was not relegated merely to interior design but was used for significant structures, such as palaces and tombs. One of its fundamental tenets is that there is a continuous flow of energy between us and our environment that can promote both physical and mental health. In this context, feng shui is one of the best ways to understand the concept of qi and how it affects health. Chinese medicine scholar-practitioner Michael Stanley-Baker recalled in a podcast interview that his Chinese medicine teacher said sleeping under a roof beam would make one prone to heart attacks. Similarly, placing your bed, couch, or desk under a beam is also thought to cause depression. It is easy to follow the logic of how sleeping or spending significant time under a lowered structure can induce feelings of oppression or claustrophobia and affect the energy of your living space.

You may be pleasantly surprised, or even astonished, to discover that there are some preliminary studies validating feng shui's effects on physical and mental health! One study in particular examined psychological and physiological responses in different feng shui indoor environments. The results showed that a room with feng shui consideration had a more positive heart rate variability and profile of mood states. From this, it was inferred that indoor spaces using feng shui principles produced more positive emotions and that they were perceived as more comfortable environments, thus proving that feng shui principles are, to a certain extent, scientific.

A 2021 randomized, double-blind study split 134 participants into three groups and gave some people recommendations for how to modify their bedrooms using feng shui principles, with those recommendations tailored according to the layout of their individual rooms. Participants who incorporated feng shui principles into their sleeping environment reported a significantly positive effect on sleep quality.

Following are some recommended feng shui principles you can incorporate into your environment to help improve mental health, especially depression.

1. The house should be well-lit and filled with sunlight. Sufficient light makes people feel positive and active whereas low-light environments are full of negative energy.

2. Avoid dark, heavy colors when decorating, as well as cool colors if prone to depression. Warm colors, such as beige, which provide a sense of warmth and calm, are best.

3. If you're looking for a new home, choose one that is square—a well-known feng shui taboo is a triangular or irregularly shaped home.

4. Do not place beds, sofas, or desks directly under a roof beam.

5. Do not spend all day in a small room, such as a bedroom; your living room should be spacious.

6. Add live plants, flowers, or a small fish tank to infuse a room with qi and vitality.

7. Beds on an upper floor should not be placed above a chandelier (in a lower room). This can negatively affect mental health and digestion. A chandelier should be replaced with a ceiling light.

8. Burn incense with warming qualities, such as mugwort, Chinese cinnamon, and Chen Pi, to dispel negative energy.

Conclusion

If you are suffering from depression, you may also want to explore chapter 6, Anxiety, and chapter 4, Insomnia, which have some overlap with depression in terms of patterns and treatment (this is also recognized in Western medicine, as a significant percentage of those with depression also experience symptoms of anxiety).

In the next chapter, we'll see that the distinction between depression and anxiety can sometimes be as little as whether you have the energy to respond to stressful situations. Let's explore this more in the following pages.

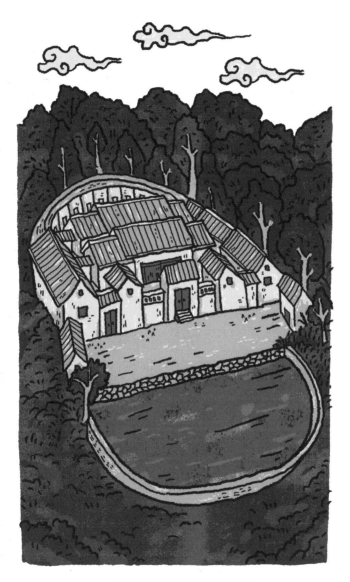

Feng shui used for placement of important
buildings in ancient China

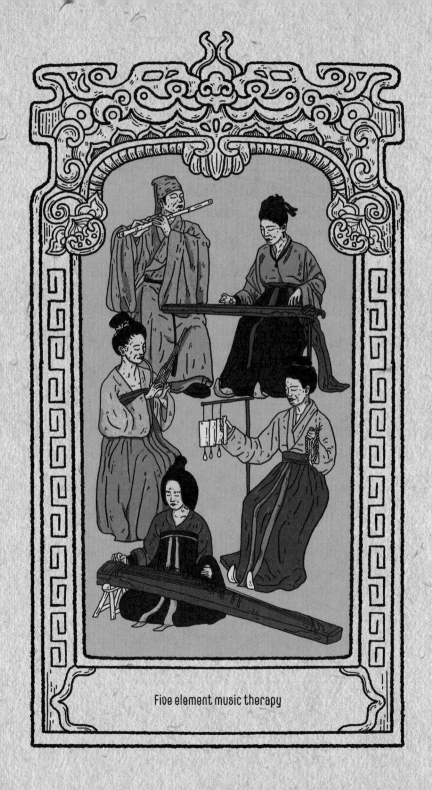

Five element music therapy

CHAPTER 6

ANXIETY

Few mental health disorders respond to Chinese medicine treatments as well as anxiety, and few conditions illustrate Chinese medicine's individualized approach better—instead of the Western mono-drug approach to sedating generalized anxiety, traditional Chinese medicine offers precise categorizations of anxiety to articulate the exact patterns of symptoms you may experience, as well as an impressive arsenal of formulas that specifically address each pattern. Given the intensity of physical response that often accompanies anxiety, special attention should be given to physiological symptoms. This chapter includes expansive recommendations on herbal formulas, several protocols for acupressure and self-massage, some beneficial teas for anxiety, as well as music therapy protocols featured in clinical studies.

An Historian's Overview of Anxiety in Traditional Chinese Medicine

The concept and condition of anxiety have been discussed in traditional Chinese medicine since the fourth century BCE. The condition, associated with a cluster of related conditions such as chu 怵 (worry), kong 恐 (fear), and jingji 驚悸 (panic), was mentioned in the early Daoist text *Zhuangzi*, as well as in medical texts such as *Inner Classic of the Yellow Emperor*. Anxiety, like a host of other emotional disorders, is understood in the Chinese medical tradition as arising from imbalances in qi due to either blocked or disordered functioning of Organs or the communicative pathways between these Organs. Specific Organs associated with the emotion of fear, which can become anxiety, are the Kidney and Lung. The Suwen holds that the five Organs, through their interaction, have an effect on the five types of qi, and this generates the various emotions, including anxiety.

Anxiety is understood as harming the spirit and the Heart and leading to a fear greater and more sustained than what we normally experience in daily life. (The Suwen also holds that anxiety harms the Lung, specifically.) Such emotions become pathological when they become overabundant or overly intense. Heightened emotion can lead to anxiety and a variety of similar pathological states. Kong (fear) is understood as one of the Five Emotions that can become imbalanced and lead to disorder.

The Heart is a key Organ that can be harmed by anxiety, according to the *Lingshu Jing*, which can then also create additional disorders and illness in the person suffering from anxiety. Numerous texts describe a host of physical symptoms that can be caused by anxiety, such as tightness in the chest, heart palpitations, abdominal pain and fullness, trembling, and the feeling of heat. These symptoms are attributed to qi being blocked from its proper movement between Organs, which leads to deficiencies, as well as the characteristic hesitation and inability to act that accompanies anxiety.

Imbalances of qi connected to dysfunction of the Organs that lead to anxiety can have direct physical causes as well, such as a poor diet or unbalanced or excessive activities connected to situational or lifestyle features. Anxiety can also emerge due to unresolved emotional imbalances created by related disorders, in this way appearing as a secondary disorder. Excessive heat can also cause anxiety and other disorders arising from emotional imbalance.

A number of traditional medical texts from ancient China discuss the cluster of anxiety concepts. In the earliest layer of medical texts, such as the Suwen and *Lingshu Jing* sections of the *Inner Classic of the Yellow Emperor*, we find an association between severe fear and anxiety and the heat created by excessive yang—a feature of qi that can be brought about through intensity, energy, heightened states of emotion, and other things marked by an energetic or frenetic character. Engaging in overly energetic activities, including excessive labor, can also bring this about.

Zhang Jiebin (1563–1640), the famous Ming dynasty physician, attributed anxiety to differential operation of four Organs (zang 臟), specifically the Heart, Spleen, Liver, and Kidney. The qi of the Heart becomes insufficient due to imbalance and misconnection with the other Organs, which directly leads to anxiety and its particular physical effects of heart palpitations. To address anxiety, according to Zhang, treatment must aim to both increase qi as well as nourish the Heart and spirit (shen), which also helps regularize the Organs.

The Suwen also focuses on the opposition of contrary emotions, holding that joy overcomes anxiety. Wu Kun (1551–1620), another famous Ming dynasty physician of the Xin'an School, added that anxiety both overcomes and is overcome by particular emotions—anxiety overcomes anger and is, in turn, overcome by joy. Thus, a focus on generating joy can help treat anger. There are, of course, numerous ways joy can be generated. The Suwen's response points to, among other solutions, self-cultivation and the reduction of desires. In Chinese medicine, there is no doubt that treating and soothing anxiety is of utmost important to the overall health of the sufferer. As the Suwen says, "If cravings and desire have no limits, if anxiety and suffering find no end, the essence qi will be destroyed."

Anxiety is also discussed in a host of philosophical texts in the Chinese tradition, including the *Zhuangzi* (c. third century BCE). In that text, anxiety (chu 怵) is understood as a result of changing circumstances and the difficulty the mind has adjusting to the inevitable changes of the world. The *Zhuangzi* offers the possibility of moving beyond such anxiety by coming to accept and, ultimately, delight in the continual changes of nature, a state we achieve through proper reflection and recognition of our ability to shift our perspective about the world from one of rigidity and resistance to one of flexibility and acceptance of change.

A Clinician's Approach to Anxiety in Traditional Chinese Medicine

There are a number of classical Chinese medical terms used to describe what we would call "anxiety" in modern times: generally, a feeling of threat, worry, and overwhelming fear. Each of these categorizations typically has its own corresponding treatment. Primary among these is the term "vexation" (fan 煩), which is a compelling image. The shape on the left, huo 火, depicts fire, and the right part refers to tou 頭, or head, in traditional Chinese. Thus, vexation is likened to a fire next your head—an apt description of an overwhelming heat-y feeling that can include mental irritability and restlessness. As we have seen, yin and yang are always in communication, so this fiery image also has a watery counterpart with an equally picturesque name: Ben Tun 奔豚, or Running Piglet.

Running Piglet defines a sudden rushing sensation that ascends to the chest and throat and a panicky feeling. In classical texts, this is attributed to fright (jing 驚). In the lower portion of this character we find the character for ma 馬, or horse, in traditional Chinese. A horse exemplifies a parasympathetic state when it is grazing, with its head and belly loose and relaxed. But, if it is startled, the horse will raise its head and burst into a gallop. This exemplifies the gesture of the body activating its defenses described as the surface of the body: The body gathers resources and pushes them out to the periphery to meet a perceived threat. The deepest center in the body is the Kidney, which represents the Water phase. Fear is the emotion attributed to Water. Thus, we could say that the mobilization of fear draws Kidney Water resources up and out to the upper and outer areas of the body. That is why fear, fright, and panic, which can lead to extremes of anxiety, are often associated with rapid breathing, increased heart rate, palpitations, and intrusive thoughts. In modern terms, we might associate these patterns with hyperarousal of the sympathetic nervous system (the fight-or-flight mode).

Another important term related to anxiety is zao 躁 (agitation). Compared to vexation, agitation is more like a *physical* feeling of restlessness, which can also be an aspect of anxiety. This is usually a response to heat in the body. Heat is often derived from any bodily hyperactivity—even conditions like fevers, physical and mental overwork, or chronic inflammation can be described as sources of heat that might lead to agitation.

Blood Deficiency can also be associated with anxiety. Blood is an important component of the nourishing, moistening, and warming functions of the body. An ample circulation is a sign of robust vitality and is indicated by the fullness, color, and warmth of the body. Cold hands and feet, for example, can indicate that the circulation is not dynamic enough to promote circulation to the tips of the toes and fingers (the farthest points from the Heart). Likewise, if the Blood cannot move up and out, it will also fail to nourish the brain, the hair, and the face. Poor memory, diminished concentration, anxiety, pallor, and dry skin and hair are all signs of Blood Deficiency. On the emotional level, anything that causes us to constrict and withdraw can contribute to these patterns.

The classical texts differentiate many causes and syndromes for anxiety. This allows us to treat each pattern with great specificity rather than a single sedating approach. It also means we can learn about our personal triggers and circumstances, and potentially adapt our lifestyle to ease anxiety.

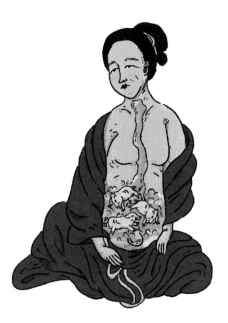

Running Piglets

Causes of Anxiety: Chinese Medicine Patterns

The most basic aspect of pattern differentiation in Chinese medicine is distinguishing excess patterns from deficient patterns.

Excess patterns are associated with the stagnation of qi, and sometimes Blood in anxiety. Qi Stagnation can give rise to feelings of "stuckness" on both emotional and physical levels, typically evidenced by pain below the ribs, tension in the neck, irritability, and headaches. Blood stasis, on the other hand, has more significant fixed and stabbing pain, and will often also affect the menses, with abdominal cramps, clots in the menstrual blood, and more labile emotions.

Deficient patterns include some forms of vexation (see chapter 4, Insomnia, and its discussion of Deficient Vexation, for example), and the Running Piglet pattern just discussed. One of Dr. Leon Hammer's most significant insights about this relates to the recurrence of the many unknowns in our lives as we grow and change. Any way in which we feel at a loss to face that fear and act can be the result of a deficient pattern.

We can also look at the Five Phases model to understand this. Each phase plays a role in our emotional life and growth. The table at right, based on Dr. Hammer's model in *Dragon Rises, Red Bird Flies*, offers a few examples.

Phase	*Organ*	*Trigger*	*Sample Symptoms*
Water	Kidney	Adverse experiences at birth or early in life, fear of the unknown, subtle developmental issues, constitutional factors	Chronic fatigue, fearfulness, low back soreness and pain, somnolence, lack of energy, failure to "keep up" with life's demands
Wood	Liver	Ability to advance and retreat, stress, opposition, powerful drive	Qi Stagnation, irritability, and agitation, perfectionism, fear of humiliation, pushing beyond one's energy
Fire	Heart/ Pericardium	Self-expression, communication, love, romance, creativity	Palpitations, increased heart rate, Running Piglet, social anxiety, fear of public speaking, all romantic issues (loves me, loves me not)
Earth	Spleen	Bonding, compassion, self-care, satisfaction of needs, positive regard	Digestive issues, tired, heavy feeling, feelings of lack or diminished inner resources, desire for or loss of a caregiver
Metal	Lung	Growth, maturity, autonomy, change, taking in the new, letting go of the old, grief, loss	Shortness of breath, asthma, shallow breathing, fear of change, school phobia

Each of these patterns can be viewed through a TCM-based pattern differentiation lens, such as Liver Qi Stagnation in the Wood phase, which can arise as a response to stress, like that irrepressible force meeting an immovable object mentioned previously.

Of course, some patterns also overlap. The famous formula Xiao Yao San (see page 75) treats a pattern of Liver Qi Stagnation (irritability), Spleen Qi Deficiency (loose stools), and Blood Deficiency (scanty or delayed menses, poor concentration). Likewise, communication between the Water and Fire phases could describe many of the more classical patterns of vexation and Running Piglet. For example, a patient may experience symptoms such as heart palpitations, panic attacks, and anxiety. On further questioning from a clinician, however, it may become clear that these feelings are associated with a new romantic relationship—not anxiety. It can sometimes be difficult to distinguish between excitement and anxiety for some people, especially if they have had past challenges. Nevertheless, these feelings can be further relieved with a Ben Tun formula, which combines aspects of Water, Fire, and even Metal. We will see how individual medicinals in the common anxiety formulas address different patterns.

Chapter 8 of the *Lingshu Jing* discusses syndromes related to emotions with terms that suggest that emotional influences cause a kind of overflowing response, perhaps indicating that the Organs are not creating a safe, contained space for the spirit (shen). With this in mind, the therapeutic principle engaged in treating anxiety is calming the spirit (安神). This is the most basic directive to treating anxiety and panic.

Remedies for Anxiety

Herbal Formulas for Anxiety

As there are many herbal formulas mentioned here, following is a summary chart to help you better understand which might be best for your circumstances. If you have anxiety (or anxiety with depression) and aren't sure where to start, try An Shen Ding Zhi Wan, Gui Pi Tang, or Jia Wei Xiao Yao San/Wan. These formulas are known for their wide availability and lack of side effects. The latter is by far the most popular formula in traditional Chinese medicine, with one research article estimating it comprised 33 to 45 percent of all Chinese medicine formulas sold. Its extreme popularity is a testament to its gentle but fast-acting nature, and it also happens to be one of the most clinically proven.

Once you decide on a formula, you should feel a noticeable difference in symptoms within the first week or two. If you do, take at full dosage for four weeks, after which you can discontinue it if symptoms abate, or take as needed. If you do not notice any difference in the first one to two weeks of taking the formula at full dosage, it may not be the right one for you.

Certain herbs are seen repeatedly in formulas for mental health. One combination of herbs that many formulas share is Gui Zhi and Fu Ling. Gui Zhi is cinnamon, and its most significant feature, in this case, is that it counteracts counterflow, meaning any overexpression of upward, outward energy as discussed in earlier sections. Fu Ling, or poria mushroom, is also very important because it both calms the spirit (shen) and helps transform Water while strengthening the center. Centeredness is a fundamental aspect of mental wellness: When faced with stress that challenges our stability, our resilience is measured by how readily we can regain a feeling of being fully in our center. Gui Zhi draws overwhelming feelings downward and strengthens our resilience; when paired with Fu Ling, it also calms and grounds. These two herbs are the basis of many Running Piglet and anxiety formulas.

A second combination is known as Heavy Spirit Settling herbs, and contains minerals. Long Gu and Mu Li occur quite commonly in Spirit Settling formulas. Here, subtleties of taste help explain the unique combination of functions exhibited by this pair. Salty Mu Li is a shell, so it descends into the depths of

Formula	*Indications/Differentiation*
Jia Wei Xiao Yao San/Wan (page 75)	Irritability, symptoms made worse by stress
An Shen Ding Zhi Wan (page 94)	Fatigue, mental exhaustion, fearfulness
Gui Pi Tang (page 96)	Worry, poor memory, pallor, poor appetite, loose stools
Tian Wang Bu Xin Dan (page 98)	Generalized anxiety, inflammation
Suan Zao Ren Tang (page 56)	Easily triggered, insomnia
Ben Ten (Running Piglet) (page 99)	Rushing sensation, palpitations, dizziness
Gan Mai Da Zao Tang (page 77)	Grief, Visceral Agitation, distress, uncontrollable crying, breakups
Gui Zhi Gan Cao Long Gu Mu Li Tang (page 114)	Heart related, ADHD
Gui Zhi Jia Long Gu Mu Li Tang (page 97)	Symptoms of heat above with cold below, profuse dreaming or yearning

the Water phase and helps dissolve any obstructions. Bland Long Gu ("dragon bone"—fossilized animal bone) is more earthy and grounding, helping us settle down and find structure and stability.

It should be noted, too, that many formulas for anxiety are also indicated for insomnia (see chapter 4), and these symptoms often occur together, such as when anxious thoughts disrupt sleep. Some formulas for anxiety are even discussed in chapter 5, Depression. It is worth noting that, at times, the distinction between depression and anxiety is whether you have the energy to respond to stressful situations, that is, engaging the Fire of a fight-or-flight sympathetic nervous system response, or going instead into freeze mode, as if overwhelmed by cold Water. The warming aspect of blood circulation has already been noted as well as how depletion of Blood through inhibited circulation or excessive blood loss can also be implicated in depression and anxiety through similar mechanisms. Now let's look at some specific remedies.

Jia Wei Xiao Yao San/Wan 加味消遥散 (Free and Easy Wanderer Plus)

This is the formula Xiao Yao San, included in the previous chapter on depression, with the addition of two herbs, Gardenia Fruit and Moutan Root Bark, which are cooling herbs that better balance the formula's synergistic effects (see page 57 for the remaining ingredients and their functions). This modified formula is more ideal for those with anxiety. A 2001 randomized, double-blind, placebo-controlled study found that, for mild to moderate depression with anxiety, Jia Wei Xiao Yao was as effective as sertraline (Zoloft), but its effect was felt sooner and was deemed safer and less expensive than its Western medicine counterpart. (Jia Wei) Xiao Yao San is the most popular formula in all of Chinese medicine and is an excellent generalized option for anxiety.

An Shen Ding Zhi Wan 安神定志 (Calm the Spirit and Settle Emotions Pill)

This widely available patent (standardized) remedy that, as its name implies, "calms the spirit and settles emotions," is widely researched for both ADHD and anxiety. It has an overall strengthening effect that treats a state of fatigue and mental exhaustion related to persistent anxiety.

Herb	Function	Indications
Ren Shen	Tonifies qi	Fatigue, feeling overtaxed
Fu Ling	Regulates Water	Palpitations
Fu Shen	Calms spirit (shen)	Anxiety, worry
Shi Chang Pu	Clears phlegm from Heart orifices	Confusion, difficulty thinking clearly, phobia
Yuan Zhi	Connects Heart and Kidney, stabilizes	Feelings of fear and apprehension, racing heart

Gui Zhi Gan Cao Long Gu Mu Li Tang 桂枝甘草龙骨牡蛎汤 **(Cinnamon Twig, Licorice, Dragon Bone, and Oyster Shell Decoction)**

The clause in the *Shanghanlun* for this remedy suggests that vexation and agitation can result from overstimulation, or a frightening stimulus. Along with anxiety, this formula can help those who also experience symptoms of ADHD. The four herbs in this remedy are focused on easing that anxiety directly and are also useful for concentration and focus.

Herb	Function	Indications
Gui Zhi	Harmonizes yang and moves qi through the chest	Anxiety with a stuffy feeling in the chest, palpitations
Gan Cao	Harmonizes and grounds sensation	Feeling unstable
Long Gu	Sedates and calms	Fright, palpitations, stirring feelings
Mu Li	Relaxes and promotes descent (interoception)	Racing thoughts, fear, confusion

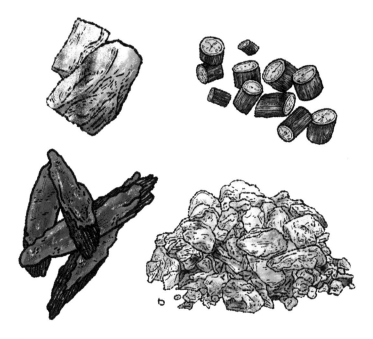

Gui Pi Tang 归脾汤 (Restore the Spleen Decoction)

Another widely available remedy, Gui Pi Tang, treats signs of Spleen Qi Deficiency and Heart Blood Deficiency, so there will be symptoms of fatigue, low voice, and shortness of breath combined with anxiety, worry, palpitations, and poor memory.

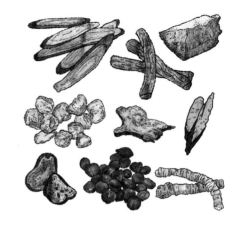

Herb	Function	Indications
Ren Shen	Tonifies qi and fluids	Fatigue
Huang Qi	Tonifies qi (adaptogen)	Low voice, shortness of breath, diminished immunity
Bai Zhu	Tonifies Spleen	Abdominal bloating, poor appetite
Fu Ling	Regulates Water, calms spirit	Fear, apprehension, need to urinate
Suan Zao Ren	Calms spirit	Anxiety, poor memory, insomnia from worry
Long Yan Rou	Nourishes Heart Blood	Poor concentration, anxiety, nervous agitation
Mu Xiang	Moves qi in the middle, supports Earth function	Fullness in the chest and abdomen, stuffiness
Zhi Gan Cao	Harmonizes	Stress
Dang Gui	Tonifies Blood	Poor memory, fatigue, pale skin, easily cold
Yuan Zhi	Connects Heart and Kidney	Anxiety, fear, apprehension

Gui Zhi Jia Long Gu Mu Li Tang 桂枝加龍骨牡蠣湯 (Cinnamon Twig Decoction Plus Dragon Bone and Oyster Shell)

Gui Zhi Tang as a stand-alone formula is indicated for vexation, especially when there are feelings of heat effusion causing discomfort. Adding Long Gu and Mu Li creates a new formula with even more potent calming action, first appearing in Zhang Zhongjing's *Essential Prescriptions of the Golden Cabinet*. It strengthens the body by restraining hyperactivity while settling the spirit and inducing calm. Feelings of cold in the groin and heat in the chest are signs to take this formula, as well as profuse yearning or longing, or dreams that leave you feeling unrested.

Herb	Function	Indications
Gui Zhi	Harmonizes yang activity	Sweating, palpitations, anxious thoughts
Bai Shao	Astringes and nourishes yin containment	Tension, lack of control, premature ejaculation
Sheng Jiang	Warms and effuses healthy internal warmth	Feeling cold but sweaty
Da Zao	Nourishes and strengthens the body	Fatigue, excessive dreaming
Zhi Gan Cao	Harmonizes and centers	Instability, palpitations
Long Gu	Sedates and calms	Agitation, impulsivity
Mu Li	Relaxes and descends	Tension

Tian Wang Bu Xin Dan 天王補心丹 (Heavenly King Tonify the Heart Special Pills)

丹 is a special term for a honey pill, and this formula is widely available in the form of tea pills (also known as wan). It is also one of the most important remedies for anxiety. Its true origins are shrouded in mystery, but it has a long history. This formula treats worry, anxiety, and hypervigilance as well as heart palpitations, shortness of breath, racing heartbeat, and other signs of autonomic dysregulation.

Herb	Function	Indications
Sheng Di Huang **Tian Men Dong** **Mai Men Dong** **Xuan Shen**	Nourishes yin fluids, nutritive	Restlessness, dry throat and mouth, night sweats
Wu Wei Zi	Calms spirit (shen)	Overthinking
Bai Zi Ren	Calms spirit, nourishes Heart Blood	Poor memory, difficulty concentrating
Suan Zao Ren	Calms spirit, nourishes Liver Blood	Excessive dreaming, wandering thoughts
Dang Gui	Moves and nourishes Blood	Pallor, dryness, brittle nails
Long Yan Rou	Nourishes Liver Blood	Poor memory, difficulty focusing
Dan Shen	Strengthens Heart qi and Blood	Palpitations, insomnia
Fu Ling	Strengthens Spleen, calms spirit	Insomnia palpitations due to phlegm, or water metabolism
Yuan Zhi	Connects Heart and Kidney	Restlessness, palpitations with anxiety, disorientation
Jie Geng	Opens chest, circulates qi	Chest congestion
Zhu Sha	Sedates and calms spirit	Restlessness, irritability

Suan Zao Ren Tang 酸枣仁汤 **(Sour Jujube Seed Decoction)**

This formula, recommended as an insomnia remedy in chapter 4, also treats a type of anxiety called Deficient Vexation, an easily triggered state of restlessness.

Herb	*Function*	*Indications*
Suan Zao Ren	Strengthens Liver Blood, calms spirit (shen)	Inability to sleep, excessive dreaming
Fu Ling	Calms spirit	Fright, palpitations
Gan Cao	Tonifies qi and yin, harmonizes	Feeling ungrounded or unresourced
Zhi Mu	Nourishes Kidney, clears deficient heat, calms Heart	Tension, heat, nervous system inflammation
Chuan Xiong	Circulates Blood, alleviates depression	Stuck feelings, fixed ideas

Ben Tun 奔豚 **(Running Piglet Formulas)**

Formulas that combine Gui Zhi and Fu Ling to address Running Piglet include the following:

- Fu Gui Ling Zhi Gan Cao Da Zao Tang (Gui Ling Cao Zao Tang)

- Fu Gui Ling Zhi Bai Zhu Gan Cao Tang (Gui Ling Zhu Gan Tang)

- Fu Gui Ling Zhi Wu Wei Zi and Gan Cao (Gui Ling Wu Wei Gan Cao Tang)

These formulas are suitable for fright and panic—in other words, symptoms such as the feelings of fluttering and palpitations in the abdomen or chest, with a sensation of air rushing upward. Although important in the traditional Chinese medicine arsenal, these formulas may not be widely available in patent (standardized) form.

Ling Gui Cao ZaoTang 苓桂草棗湯 (Poria, Cinnamon Twig, Licorice, and Jujube Decoction)

This formula is especially indicated for feelings of anxiety with a pulsating feeling in the abdomen and palpitations. This could also be like the butterflies you feel in your stomach when you are anxious or apprehensive. This formula also helps when an abundance of thoughts overwhelms you, making you feel a little out of control.

Herb	Function	Indications
Fu Ling	Calms spirit	Fluttering sensations, dizziness, recurrent thoughts
Gui Zhi	Harmonizes yang and moves qi through the chest	Palpitations, sweating
Zhi Gan Cao	Benefits Earth, harmonizes herbs	Feeling ungrounded
Da Zao	Nourishes qi and Blood	Fatigue

Gui Ling Wu Wei Gan Cao Tang 桂苓五味甘草湯 (Cinnamon Twig, Poria, Schisandra, and Licorice Decoction)

This formula alleviates very specific symptoms that could be called performance anxiety or stage fright. Alongside the palpitations and anxiety, there might be numbness in the extremities, tunnel vision, a need to urinate, blushing or red face, and feeling hot.

Herb	Function	Indications
Gui Zhi	Warms yang and descends counterflow	Palpitations, red face
Fu Ling	Calms spirit, regulates Water metabolism	Frequent urination
Wu Wei Zi	Astringes, calms, gathers spirit	Numbness, tingling
Gan Cao	Harmonizes	Feeling uneasy

Gui Ling Zhu Gan Tang 苓桂朮甘湯 (Poria, Cinnamon Twig, Atractylodes, and Licorice Decoction)

This formula especially treats dizziness and trembling, with feelings of abdominal fullness, possibly difficult urination, thirst without a dry mouth, shortness of breath, feelings like air rushing upward as in a state of panic, and palpitations. This formula focuses on establishing centeredness and clarity by promoting Water metabolism.

Herb	Function	Indications
Fu Ling	Calms spirit (shen), drains Water	Dizziness, trembling, urinary issues
Gui Zhi	Promotes yang movement, warms	Palpitations, uprushing feeling
Bai Zhu	Strengthens Earth, eliminates bloating and fullness	Bloating, abdominal fullness
Zhi Gan Cao	Harmonizes all herbs	Feeling uneasy

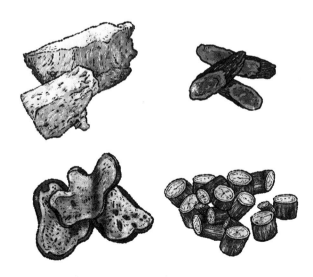

Gan Mai Da Zao Tang 甘麥大棗湯 (Licorice Wheat Jujube Decoction)

This classical Chinese formula treats pervasive, overwhelming feelings of anxiety, restlessness, loss of control, unmanageable crying, and frequent yawning and sighing. This is also useful in states of grief and depression.

Herb	Function	Indications
Fu Xiao Mai	Settles emotions	Visceral Agitation: feeling overwhelmed by emotion and grief, sadness, melancholy
Gan Cao	Centers and grounds	Instability, difficulty restraining tears and emotion
Da Zao	Nourishes qi and Blood	Nervous exhaustion and feeling overwhelmed

Tea and the Importance of GABA for Anxiety

Undoubtedly, the most popular health drink in the world and the second most popular beverage after water, tea (here, and throughout the book, defined as the beverage made from the leaves of the *Camellia sinensis* plant) is a drink often consumed for its cognitive effects, whether to impart a mental boost or to slow us down. A pot of pu'er tea (a tea often considered the richest in health benefits due to its fermentation, and supported by an abundance of clinical studies) also happens to be the most essential part of my daily wellness routine. Although tea originated in China and has been a ubiquitous part of Chinese culture for millennia, in recent years, younger generations in China have adopted new forms of tea drinking, including making tea in clay teapots over a charcoal fire at their dining room table. This rustic way of preparing tea (some even roast fruits and snacks over the charcoal while waiting for the water to boil!) has become such a popular trend that multiple municipal health departments throughout China issued warning statements about carbon monoxide poisoning for those without proper ventilation.

This latest Chinese trend is part of a renewed interest in tea that has seen China's national beverage emerge as one of the main symbols of a slower pace of life, and teas such as pu'er have become one of the most prized collectibles in Asia. "Aged pu'er is seen as a 'slow beverage,' used to counterbalance the rapid pace of modernity," according to Jinghong Zhang's book, *Puer Tea: Ancient Caravans and Urban Chic*. Many people also view tea preparation as a grounding or meditative practice, which can provide a sense of peace during times of stress or anxiety. There is, indeed, symbolism and a ceremonial or ritualistic component of drinking tea—it was important in temples, where Buddhist monks drank it to refresh their mind and assist in

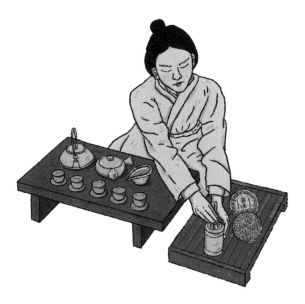

meditation, as expressed in the saying "Tea and Ch'an (Zen) Buddhism have the same flavor" or "cha chan yi wei."

However, tea also possesses unique phytochemicals that give it a very different feel from any other beverage, including coffee. If you're prone to anxiety, coffee or energy drinks can be too stimulating. Clinical studies confirm that the caffeine equivalent of five cups of coffee can induce panic attacks in a large proportion of patients with panic disorder, and increases anxiety in panic disorder patients. Although tea also contains caffeine—each cup of tea is usually about a quarter to a third the caffeine of an equivalent cup of coffee—tea's other phytochemicals include the amino acid L-theanine, which can work synergistically with caffeine to provide a calm wakefulness and alertness. L-theanine has been shown to significantly increase activity in the alpha frequency band—in brain waves that indicate that

consumption of L-theanine relaxes the mind without inducing drowsiness.

All teas also contain at least a modest amount of GABA, or gamma-aminobutyric acid, a neurotransmitter that can induce relaxation and diminish anxiety. GABA was long thought to be unable to cross the blood-brain barrier, but recently, multiple accounts have concluded that substantial amounts of GABA can cross the blood-brain barrier. This validates the feeling tea drinkers have observed for centuries—that drinking tea induces a remarkable sense of focused calmness, thanks to the phytochemicals in tea, which reach our brain as well as our gut.

The teas generally thought to be high in GABA include white tea, oolong, and raw pu'er, but since the 1980s, tea growers in Japan, China, and elsewhere have developed special GABA-enriched teas, known simply as GABA teas, through an oxygen-free fermentation process. Several studies have tested GABA oolong teas, in particular, with an Australian study concluding that its consumption led to a significant decrease in the immediate stress score and a significant improvement in heart rate variability. These findings indicate that making tea a part of your daily wellness routine can reduce your anxiety and help you enter a state of calm focus.

If you aren't familiar with tea, or never found a tea you truly enjoyed, I recommend pu'er or oolong as a wonderful place to start. These two tea types have extremely delicious and interesting flavor profiles, with my favorites being ripe pu'er, Tieguanyin, and Zhang Ping Shui Xian. The latter two are oolongs with a fragrant, floral aroma and a honey quality without any sugar. Zhang Ping Shui Xian is also known for having a creaminess of texture. Ripe pu'er is easily my favorite drink, and given its full body and rich flavor profile, is a delicious option, especially if you're accustomed to coffee or enjoy drinks like Scotch. I've recently discovered Laochatou, or "old tea heads," a special category of ripe pu'er tea nuggets that have a smooth, malty taste and are a by-product of the ripe pu'er fermentation process. I'd also strongly suggest staying away from bagged tea and jumping straight into whole leaf tea (pu'er often comes in compressed cakes, so I don't use the term "loose leaf," which can be confusing because the leaves are not loose). Good-quality tea leaves can be re-steeped many times throughout the day, with second or third steepings often considered superior to the first steep, and if calculated by the cup, usually end up less expensive than bagged tea. Or, if you hate tea leaves, check out tea resins, a rare form of instant pu'er tea that originated in ancient China and are available online through The Eastern Philosophy.

Making Pu'er Tea

Since most readers may not be familiar with pu'er tea, instructions for making it, using mini tea cakes, are as follows:

1. Remove the paper wrapping from the tea cake.

2. Place the mini tea cake into a cup, then pour boiling water directly over the tea.

3. Tea connoisseurs often prefer to give compressed tea cakes an initial 10-second steep to help loosen the leaves, then pour out the water and refill the cup.

4. For **ripe** pu'er tea, steep the tea for 1 minute, then strain out the leaves.

5. For **raw** pu'er tea, steep the tea for 30 to 45 seconds, then strain out the leaves. This is my preference; you may prefer your tea more or less strong, but these steeping times ensure your tea will not become bitter through oversteeping.

6. Enjoy your tea. Increase the steeping time by 15 to 30 seconds each time you re-steep your used tea leaves. The leaves should be discarded, or composted, at the end of the day to avoid microbial overgrowth.

For pu'er tea resins:

Place one resin in a large teapot. Add hot water (boiling water is best, but not essential). Once the resin melts, stir or shake as needed and enjoy.

Acupressure and Self-Massage for Anxiety

Press the following points for a few minutes throughout the day. You can use your pointer finger, middle finger, an acupressure stick, or, in a pinch, the eraser end of a pencil. You do not need to press hard to stimulate these points. Practiced regularly, or even just as needed, these points will help reduce anxiety.

Auricular (Ear) Massage

This exercise does not target one specific point but rather is a self-massage exercise to stimulate multiple points along the ear that can calm and soothe anxiety.

1. Rub your hands together to warm them.

2. Massage the ear from front to back with your fingers, lightly grasping the posterior ear and gently pulling it forward 5 to 10 times.

3. Softly holding the helix, the prominent rim defining the ear, with your thumb and index finger, massage all the way from the ear apex (highest point of the ear) to the earlobe until the whole ear feels warm.

4. Massage the earlobe by gently pulling the lobe down and slightly outward 5 to 10 times.

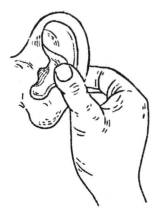

Sanyinjiao 三阴交 (Three Yin Crossing)

This point is so-called because it is where all three yin channels on the inside of the leg converge. It is easy to locate by finding a slight, often sensitive depression, about a hand's width above the medial malleolus (the small prominent bone on the inner side of the ankle at the end of the tibia). Research has shown that this point is close to a nerve bundle that, indeed, has three trajectories and exerts influence on the rest of the body through the afferent pathways and the central nervous system. It is well known for its spirit-calming effect, emphasizing the calm, collected, restorative aspect of the Spleen Earth in union with the Kidney and Liver. In addition to calming anxiety, this point can ease pain. It is especially helpful for menstrual cramps.

Apply gentle pressure on Sanyinjiao (Spleen 6) until the soreness subsides.

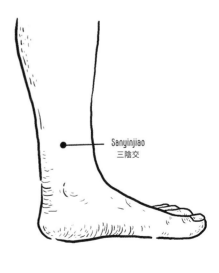

Sanyinjiao
三陰交

Heart Meridian Points

In Chinese medicine theory, there are a number of meridians, or channels, on the body strongly related to anxiety, and the points along the Heart Meridian are of particular importance, often used by acupuncturists to relieve anxiety in patients. You can achieve the same effect by stimulating these same points via acupressure. In general, points below the elbows and knees, known as the Transporting Points, are both accessible and potent. The renowned psychiatrist turned Chinese medicine practitioner Dr. Leon Hammer referred to this group as the hypnotic points in reference to their calming effect. Among them is HT 7 Shenmen 神门 (Spirit Gate), a point that eases anxiety and worry.

On the Heart Meridian, especially in this part of the meridian along the wrist, gently but firmly press the thumb along the palmar surface of the wrist, from just above the wrist crease toward the palm and little finger to engage a group of points in the Heart Meridian.

LV 3 Tai Chong 太冲 (Great Rushing)

On the foot, there is a point between the first and second toes that also offers a potent channel for addressing anxiety, and it has been extensively studied for its ability to reduce hypertension. As the source point of the Liver channel, it acts upon the associated Organ directly. It promotes a feeling of ease by nourishing and softening rigidity and alleviating tension. If you feel stressed and have pain in the flanks and ribs, this is a point to use. The point is located between the first and second metatarsals on the top of the foot, at the slight depression where the two metatarsals meet.

Use a small rotating, pressing motion on LV 3 Tai Chong for just a few minutes to activate it. You should feel immediately relaxed and less emotionally tense. You can do this exercise as many times per day as needed.

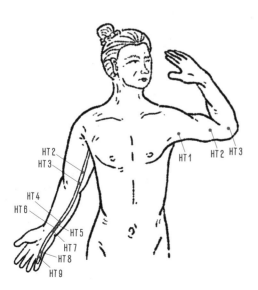

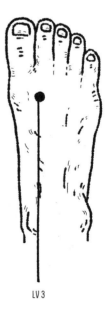

LV 3

Five Element Music Therapy for Anxiety

Anxiety can be a symptom associated with multiple patterns and Organ systems, the most common patterns being Heart and Kidney Yin Deficiency; Heart and Liver Qi Stagnation with Fire, Liver, and Kidney Yin Deficiency; and Heart and Spleen Blood Deficiency. Therefore, a range of Five Element music notes can be suitable for anxiety, particularly "music with stable rhythm instead of obvious up and down changes." The most therapeutic Five Element music for anxiety falls into Gong (Spleen/Earth), Zhi (Heart/Fire), Jue (Liver/Wood), and Yu (Kidney/Water) keys.

Two controlled studies have investigated Five Element music's effects on easing anxiety, both concluding that it was effective or significantly effective. One study evaluated Five Element music therapy on the anxiety and insomnia of medical staff during the COVID-19 outbreak, as they were isolated and under substantial pressure. Eighty-eight study participants played music for thirty minutes per day over the course of sixteen days. According to the study, anxiety and insomnia scores significantly decreased, with results showing that "both general music and Five-Element music can alleviate the anxiety and insomnia of medical staff, but the Five-Element music intervention is more effective." The study mentioned that Gong-note music was played for anxiety, including the track "Shimian Maifu" (other Gong music includes "Good Night," "Idle Life," and "Malan Flowers Bloom").

A smaller controlled study from 2018 out of Beijing Normal University observed the effect of Five Element music therapy on patients with anxiety mixed with depression. Patients in the control group were given conventional Western (pharmaceutical) medicine treatment, and patients in the observation group were given Five Element music therapy. Depression scores of both groups decreased after treatment, and the decrease was more obvious in the Five Element music group. The total effective rate of clinical treatment in this group was also higher than that in the control group. The study had participants select the musical track, put them in a quiet environment with a comfortable indoor temperature under full sunshine, and played music at 9 a.m. and 3 p.m. every day for thirty minutes over the course of four weeks. Some of the music mentioned included Jiangnan Silk and Bamboo Song, "Bu Bu Gao," and "Purple Bamboo Melody." You can also follow the researcher-designed protocol we detailed in chapter 4, Insomnia.

Conclusion

If you are suffering from anxiety, you may also want to explore chapter 4, Insomnia; chapter 5, Depression; and chapter 7, ADHD. These conditions have some overlap with anxiety in terms of patterns and treatment (in Western medicine, anxiety and depression are also considered comorbid conditions). Symptoms of anxiety can also manifest as feelings of restlessness common among those suffering from ADHD. Let's explore this more in the following pages.

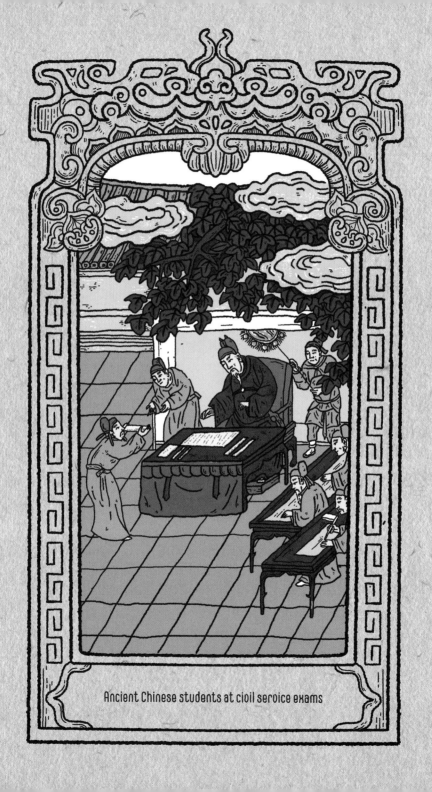

Ancient Chinese students at civil service exams

CHAPTER 7

ADHD AND LACK OF FOCUS

Did you know that Adderall and other amphetamines were discovered during the first attempts to synthesize the Chinese medicine herb Ma Huang (*Ephedra sinica*)? As mentioned in chapter 3, Ma Huang is primarily used in Chinese medicine to treat respiratory issues like asthma and bronchitis, and there are a multitude of herbs considered superior for enhancing focus and cognition, with no stimulant effects. These herbs can also calm the body and mind, strengthen memory, clear brain fog, and even help reverse cognitive decline.

Attention deficit hyperactivity disorder (ADHD) may be a relatively new term, but you may be surprised to learn that Chinese medicine has a long tradition of treating inability to focus, thanks to its storied history of the Imperial Exams, a multiple-round examination system for civil service candidates, which originated during the Sui dynasty (581–618 CE). These exams were incredibly difficult, taking place over the course of many years, ultimately with only a 1 percent passing rate. This was the origin of the concept of meritocracy, and a class of elites was created based on merit only, as the exams were open to men from any class and there were even measures in place to ensure fairness, such as using numbers instead of names and having all answers recopied to prevent handwriting recognition of ancient "nepo babies." As a result, education became firmly cemented as the most highly valued asset in ancient Chinese society, with an enduring cultural legacy. Many herbal formulas to improve focus came to prominence as a result of this rigorous examination system, including some of the subsequent recommendations here.

The Chinese medicine approach to ADHD represents a completely different approach to the Western medical one, and you won't experience the intense stimulant feeling or any of the debilitating side effects, such as lack of appetite, extreme fatigue, anxiety, insomnia, or the nightly crash, followed by a sometimes intensely depressed mood. There are also the lesser known side effects that can accompany long-term stimulant use, such as jaw clenching and teeth grinding, hair loss, skin problems, and, most alarmingly, gray matter abnormalities in the brain.

Instead of repeatedly pushing your body to its limits, sapping energy reserves that often feel unsustainable and building a tolerance to dopamine production, the methods in this chapter take a gentler, more nourishing approach to "supplement deficiency" and "reduce excess." Let's take a closer look.

An Historian's Overview of ADHD and Lack of Focus in Traditional Chinese Medicine

Attention deficit hyperactivity disorder (ADHD) is recognized in modern medicine as a complex neurobehavioral condition influenced by both genetic and environmental factors and affects both children and adults. It is characterized by a pattern of behaviors that includes inattention and/or hyperactivity, as well as impulsivity that does not align with the person's age or developmental standards. Although it is a relatively recently discovered condition in Western medicine, clinical observations consistent with ADHD have been recorded in Chinese medical texts for more than two millennia.

In Chinese medicine, the Kidney is regarded as the root of Prenatal Qi (vital life force); it plays a significant role in the formation of marrow, bones, teeth, and brain, thus, brain-based disorders are considered to be Kidney-related. According to one of the oldest Chinese medical texts, *Inner Classic of the Yellow Emperor*, at the age of seven in females and eight in males, the Kidney qi becomes abundant. This period is also associated with the natural replacement of the initial teeth and an increase in hair growth, which are indicative of brain development; as a result, this age range is believed to be the onset time for the emergence of ADHD. In the *Inner Classic*, attention deficit is identified as a yin disorder (Yang Deficiency and/or Yin Excess), described as if the Heart lacks support, the spirit (shen) has no place to return to, and one's thoughts find no ground to rest upon. The *Inner Classic* also details hyperactivity symptoms associated with yang disorder (Yang Excess and/or Yin De-

ficiency), characterized by behaviors such as climbing to high places, discarding one's clothing, running about frenetically, speaking nonsensical words, hurling insults at others regardless of one's relationship to them, and displaying a lack of desire to eat.

During the Song dynasty (960–1279), the civil service examination system became dominant for selecting individuals for governmental positions. The system's evaluation process was based on people's knowledge of the Confucian classics and command of certain literary skills, which gave rise to a new literati class and the class of literate physicians. Given the importance of scholarly pursuits, literate physicians placed greater emphasis on the treatment of attention deficit hyperactivity disorder due to its potential to impair educational performance and social interactions within academic environments. One of the most influential literate physicians in the Song era, Yan Jizhong, documented Qian Yi's Six-Ingredient Rehmannia Pill in his *Craft of Medicinal Treatment for Childhood Disease Patterns*. Drawing inspiration from the third-century herbal formula Kidney Qi Pill, Qian Yi, an esteemed pediatrician of the eleventh century, posited that a deficiency in Kidney qi was the fundamental component underlying the symptoms of ADHD and could be cured by the Six-Ingredient Rehmannia Pill, a variant version of the Kidney Qi Pill, which has been prescribed for centuries and remains one of the most recognized prescriptions for ADHD in Chinese medicine today.

Following the development of knowledge of modern anatomy along with Catholic missionaries in the sixteenth century, several Chinese literate physicians, such as Wang Honghan (seventh century), Wang Kentang (sixteenth century), and Zhao Xuemin (eighteenth century), began to regard symptoms related to ADHD as brain-based disorders. Based on the belief that emotional, mental, physical, and environmental factors all contribute to an individual's health, therapies during this era encompassed a range of treatments, such as Warm Gallbladder Decoction, Bupleurum Decoction Plus Dragon Bone and Oyster Shell, Left-Restoring Pill, and Spleen-Returning Decoction, as well as the use of acupuncture and massage therapy to harmonize the mind-body connection and alleviate symptoms associated with ADHD. The Warm Gallbladder Decoction (Wen Dan Tang 溫膽湯), formulated by Yao Sengyuan in the sixth century, features a significant quantity of fresh ginger aimed at warming the cold gallbladder. In twelfth-century southern China, Chen Wuze revised the decoction by reducing the amount of fresh ginger used; this adjustment transformed the original warming nature to a cooling nature. Since then, the revised Warm Gallbladder Decoction has gained popularity in China's warmer southern areas, where heat-related illnesses are more prevalent, and it has become one of the most popular remedies for ADHD-related symptoms.

A Clinician's Approach to ADHD and Lack of Focus in Traditional Chinese Medicine

ADHD is a clearly defined set of symptoms outlined in *The Diagnostic and Statistical Manual of Mental Disorders*, fifth edition, which is the standard classification of mental disorders used by mental health professionals in the United States. In Chinese medicine, the symptoms are similar to vexation and agitation as discussed elsewhere in this book. ADHD, however, can be understood through the concept of neurodiversity. This term denotes a broad range of differences in the nervous systems, brain functions, and traits that make up the whole range of human expression. That means that we do not have to view it as a disease that has to be eradicated, or even "cured." In fact, it's worth keeping in mind that many so-called "high achievers" consider symptoms of their ADHD their "superpowers," including high energy, creativity, empathy, and bouts of hyperfocus.

In conventional medicine, the most common treatment for the condition is long-term stimulant medication to manage symptoms. This also reflects the greatest weakness of the conventional model. The effects of stimulants are tough on the body and, in the last few years, there have also been periods marked by shortages and unavailability of prescriptions, making consistent symptom management even more challenging.

Chinese medicine offers a different approach that can improve the symptoms of ADHD, such as inattention, difficulty focusing, hyperfixation, impulsivity, restlessness, and hyperactivity. Because ADHD is defined as a neurodevelopmental condition, it is often identified by very proscribed (discouraged) criteria related to a typical school setting, such as talking in class, climbing on chairs, and fidgeting. However, children are not the only ones who deal with ADHD symptoms, as evidenced by the surge in ADHD diagnosis in adults. Fortunately, Chinese herbs can provide many effective solutions.

As with other patterns, in Chinese medicine, we seek to harmonize the extremes of yin and yang, realizing there are times for excitement and spontaneity and times for stillness and effort. The poles of both states are interconnected within the mind. Some behaviors benefit from strengthening reserves and boundaries, whereas others require a more strictly settling action and a decrease in energy. We describe these as "supplementing deficiency" and "reducing excess." It is a very simple issue: If there is too much, take some away, and if there is too little, add more. As we examine patterns, we will see how this plays out in the Heart.

Causes of ADHD and Lack of Focus: Chinese Medicine Patterns

In examining the basic symptoms of ADHD, we see that they are divided into inattentive aspects and hyperactive aspects, which also include impulsivity. From a traditional Chinese medicine perspective, this division fits rather neatly into our basic deficient or excess pattern. In addition, it also correlates to the patterns of vexation and agitation, similar in many respects to insomnia (see chapter 4) and anxiety (see chapter 6). All involve a spirit that is not at rest. Attention wanders when the spirit is not contained, and this can occur under the influence of heat—it is as if heat rises and carries away the spirit, inhibiting attention and focus.

When we discuss the vexation that occurs with Running Piglet (starting on page 89), there is a lack of clarity. Rather than heat flaring up, we can liken this to Water bubbling up and extinguishing the Fire of the

Heart. The bubbling sensation can also be described as palpitations or pulsations, and may produce symptoms such as dizziness or instability. These symptoms are more associated with inattention, or excess yin in the Heart. In the early texts where Running Piglet is first described, the excess of yin affecting the upper burner or Heart is described as a Water metabolism issue.

In later texts, a similar process became more prominent as an explanation for changes in the sensory function and clarity in relation to the Heart: Phlegm Misting the Orifices of the Heart. This can be more or less extreme and, in ADHD, it's the less extreme manifestation. Nevertheless, it is interesting to consider that there is a continuum that spans from a tendency toward denial to inattention to confusion to delusion and all the way to auditory or visual hallucinations. The common denominator in these conditions is a disruption of concentration and cognitive acuity. If this is further complicated by heat, restlessness and hyperactivity also result.

All of these patterns can arise in the context of a sensitive nervous system. Typically, that can be related to early life experience, or diet and lifestyle, or a combination of factors. A person with a sensitive nervous system could have a heightened openness to creative ideas, thoughts, and insights, but the same quality that creates that openness can complicate organization, timeliness, and impulse control. Over time, a person can develop anxiety about things like public speaking or structured projects. If they do not get support, this anxiety can lead to repeated failure in school or work settings. Eventually, even depression can arise in response to the exhaustion of the inner resources. This is an example of the real potential of Chinese medicine to address conditions like ADHD. Pattern recognition, and an understanding of the ecology of symptoms (i.e., a context-rich perception), can both validate a person's experience and offer relief. That's powerful medicine.

Pattern differentiation using traditional Chinese medicine diagnosis allows us to distinguish different causes and responses: different stressors in variable terrains. For example, diet can be an influence on the creation of a phlegm that clouds perception. Inhibited digestion can create excess turbid Dampness, with signs like loose stools and abdominal bloating, and then eventually affect the Heart. We can even see this through the lens of chronic inflammation and the gut microbiome and how these factors influence behavior. In fact, this is what Chinese medicine has been describing all along.

Remedies for ADHD and Lack of Focus

Herbal Formulas for ADHD and Lack of Focus

The following formulas can be taken long term or as needed to improve focus, such as during exams week. Traditional Chinese herbal patent (standardized) medicines are generally safe and this book features formulas regarded as safe and well-balanced. Look for the symptoms that match your experience, paying special attention to physical symptoms in this section. Refer to chapter 3, which provides more detail on how to take herbal formulas.

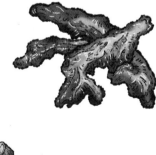

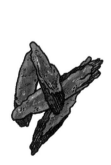

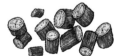

Gui Zhi Gan Cao Long Gu Mu Li Tang 桂枝甘草龙骨牡蛎汤 (Cinnamon Twig, Dragon Bone, and Oyster Shell Decoction)

Gui Zhi Gan Cao Long Gu Mu Li Tang appears in the *Shanghanlun* and specifically treats vexation and agitation. These terms account for both mental and physical symptoms defining ADHD, such as inattention and impulsivity, as well as restlessness and fidgeting.

Herb	*Function*	*Indications*
Gui Zhi	Warms and circulates qi in the chest	Inattention, lack of concentration, difficulty sustaining effort
Zhi Gan Cao	Sweetens, nourishes, provides centeredness	Ungrounded, scattered
Long Gu	Heavy minerals settle and calm	Agitation, impulsivity
Mu Li	Salty minerals settle and soften hardness	Tension

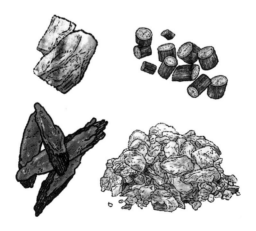

Fu Ling Gui Zhi Gan Cao Da Zao Tang 茯苓桂枝甘草大枣汤 (Poria, Cinnamon Twig, Licorice, and Jujube Decoction)

This is a formula that works with Water metabolism to treat Running Piglet syndrome. Running Piglet is a condition derived from fright, described as an uprushing feeling from the lower abdomen to the chest, and an overwhelming sense of panic. *Avoid this formula if you have digestive issues.*

Herb	Function	Indications
Fu Ling	Nourishes and calms spirit (shen), promotes Water metabolism, strengthens digestion	Uprushing sensations, palpitations, fear and fright
Gui Zhi	Warms Heart and Blood, promoting free flow	Inattention, lack of focus
Zhi Gan Cao	Sweetens, nourishes, strengthens the center	Enervation, nervousness
Da Zao	Provides food-like nourishment for Blood and Earth	Feeling ill at ease and out of resources

Huang Lian E Jiao Tang 黃蓮阿膠湯 (Coptis and Gelatin Decoction)

Huang Lian E Jiao Tang is typically used for insomnia (see chapter 4), but it both nourishes Blood and fluids as well as descends Fire, causing an intense inability to rest from the Heart back into the root, where it is embraced by the deeply nourishing resources of egg yolks and gelatin. In the Qin and Han dynasties, beef gelatin was used to make E Jiao, and it is recommended here over other forms of E Jiao. See page 58 for formula details. As most formulas do not contain egg yolk as purchased, it needs to be added after—simply stir raw egg yolks into the strained decoction when the temperature decreases. This formula may not be widely available.

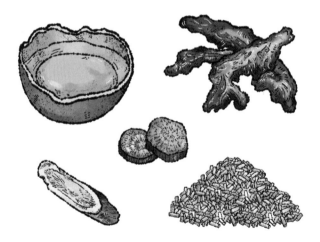

Huang Lian Wen Dan Tang 黃連溫膽湯 **(Warm Gallbladder Decoction with Coptis)**

Huang Lian Wen Dan Tang is a modification of the formula Wen Dan Tang—one of the most popular formulas for ADHD in China—and treats manifestations of heat and phlegm. Phlegm heat, especially affecting the Heart Spirit, can stoke the Fire of agitation and insomnia while creating disorientation and dizziness due to Dampness clouding the senses. The addition of Huang Lian uses the bitter taste to descend the heat harassing above and causing agitation, while the remainder of the formula supports digestion to promote healthy transformation. Use during times of extreme stress, difficulty sleeping, excessive worry, and a lack of clarity. This well-balanced formula is safe to take longer term.

Herb	Function	Indications
Huang Lian	Bitter taste descends Fire harassing the spirit (shen)	Severe agitation and impulsivity
Fu Ling **Chen Pi** **Ban Xia** **Sheng Jiang** **Gan Cao**	Promotes digestion and transformation	Phlegm, Dampness, mucus, abdominal bloating, clouded senses, confusion, poor focus
Zhu Ru	Transforms phlegm	Inattention, lack of clarity
Zhi Shi	Descends and moves qi	Fixation, impulsivity
Da Zao	Nourishes and grounds	Lack of centeredness and ease

Liu Wei Di Huang Wan 六味地黄 (Six-Ingredient Rehmannia Pill)

As noted in the historian's overview, this classical formula—itself a modification of the classical formula *Shen Qi Wan* (now more commonly called Jin Kui/Gui Shen Qi Wan)—was specifically formulated for children who were perceived as already having abundant yang energy, and so not requiring the warming effect of the herbs Gui Zhi and Fu Ling. Instead, this formula promotes fluids and stability. It is best for patients experiencing high activity levels and impulsivity, but they may also have frequent urination, agitation, hot hands and feet, and a flushed face.

Herb	Function	Indications
Shu Di Huang	Nourishes Blood and yin	Dizziness, weakness in low back or slight build
Shan Zhu Yu	Nourishes Liver and Kidney	Instability, agitation
Shan Yao	Tonifies Spleen and Kidney	Feeling ungrounded
Ze Xie	Promotes urination	Scanty, yellow urine
Mu Dan Pi	Regulates Blood heat	Feeling hot, especially hands and feet, night sweats
Fu Ling	Promotes urination, calms spirit (shen)	Agitation, urinary symptoms

Bu Nao Wan 补脑丸 (Brain Repair Pill)

As a "brain tonic," the patent formula Bu Nao Wan can provide a nourishing and calming effect to help gather thoughts and lessen impulsivity; if you have inattentive qualities that get described as spaciness and tend to be more fatigued, cold, and achy, this formula may help clear your thoughts, help you stay focused, and help you feel more attentive and engaged. It can be taken long term and also during times of high stress or increased symptoms.

Herb	Function	Indications
Suan Zao Ren	Calms spirit (shen), eliminates deficient vexation	Easily agitated, inflammation in the nervous system
Dang Gui	Tonifies Blood	Feeling slightly cold, pale skin, dry skin and nails
Hu Tao Ren	Directly supports the Brain through tonifying yang	Cold low back, slight back pain
Rou Cong Rong	Tonifies yang	Frequent urination, cold feelings
Gou Qi Zi	Tonifies Blood	Dry eyes, fatigue, pallor
Wu Wei Zi	Astringes (gathers thoughts), calms spirit	Irritability, poor concentration
Bai Zi Ren	Nourishes Heart Blood	Insomnia, poor focus, disorganized, easily distracted
Yi Zhi Ren	Astringes the Kidney, benefits essence	Frequent urination, loose stools
Tian Ma	Extinguishes Wind	Headache (whole head feels heavy), dizziness, numbness in the extremities, tremors
Hu Po	Calms spirit (shen)	Mental agitation, insomnia
Yuan Zhi	Harmonizes Heart and Kidney	Diminished awareness, erratic thought patterns
Tian Nan Xing	Dries Dampness, disperses phlegm	Dizziness, difficult breathing or cough, numbness
Tian Zhu Huang	Clears and transforms phlegm	Difficulty finding words, tics, slight tremors
Long Gu	Settles and calms spirit	Emotional stress, agitation, insomnia

Acupressure for ADHD and Lack of Focus

Practicing acupressure is itself a powerful reset for the system; taking just a few minutes to recalibrate and settle your nervous system, even without specific acupressure, can be very helpful too. For example, your breath can then lead to a practice of drawing your awareness deep into the abdomen, where stillness can be felt as a physical sensation. Gently placing your hands just below your navel and feeling the rise and fall of your abdomen with every breath will also contribute to relaxation and ease in the moment. In the age of smartphones, harnessing technology to periodically remind ourselves to do an acupressure exercise is easy.

Following are a few suggestions on some specific points to work with for relief of ADHD symptoms. First and foremost is perhaps the most vital spirit-calming point in the body: the extra point Yintang, which we have described in the chapter 4, Insomnia. Sometimes referred to as the Third Eye Point, Yintang can promote the relaxation of the forebrain, which can then enhance executive function by calming an overactive mind or overwhelming thoughts and impulses.

Small Intestine Channel

On a related note, working with points along the Small Intestine channel—found along the outside edge of the hand, from the outside of the pinky finger to the wrist crease—can be beneficial because of a few interrelated concepts.

In Chinese medicine, the Small Intestine is charged with separating the clear from the turbid. In the body, this means recognizing what is digestible and what is indigestible.

In terms of the mind, though, it helps us separate thoughts from feelings, ideas from urges, and positive from negative. In addition, the Small Intestine is the yang counterpart to the Heart within the Fire phase, so it draws away any injurious influence from the Heart-Mind.

Finally, the point Houxi SI 3—located at the small bulge when a loose fist is made—is the master point of the meridian known as the Governing Du Vessel, which has a strong relationship to the brain and nervous system because of its trajectory along the spine and centerline of the head. Yintang, just mentioned, also lies along the trajectory of the Du Vessel.

I recommend massaging these points along the side of the hand on the outer edge of the fifth metacarpal, or the side of the palm from the fingers to the wrist: from SI 3 to SI 5 in the direction of the Heart (or toward the elbow, if that makes more sense). SI 5 is adjacent to the source point of the Heart, Shen Men, so visualize these two points connecting and bring clarity to your awareness. In the Master Tung system of acupuncture, these two points are related to the Kidney, and the long metacarpal bone also represents the spine, reinforcing the nervous system settling effect of self-massage. In turn, regular use of these acupressure techniques will provide both calm and focus.

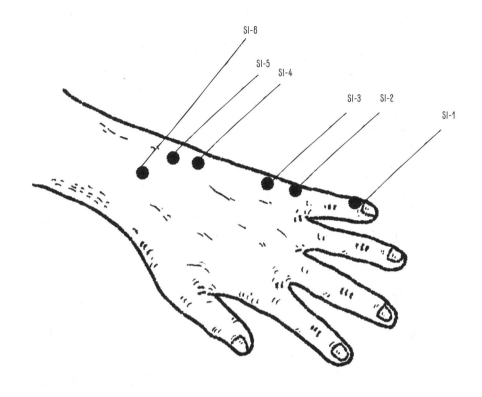

Conclusion

As mentioned in the historian's overview, another beneficial practice for ADHD is massage therapy, such as tui na, which we introduced in chapter 4, Insomnia. If you are suffering from ADHD, you may also want to explore chapter 4 as well as chapter 6, Anxiety, and chapter 8, Brain Fog, which have some significant overlap in terms of patterns and treatment to ADHD. Let's explore one of these, brain fog, in the following chapter.

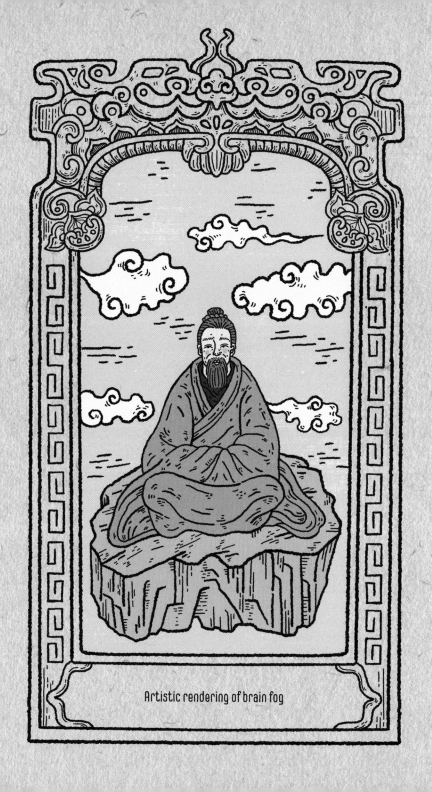
Artistic rendering of brain fog

CHAPTER 8

BRAIN FOG

Brain fog is a condition that has increased dramatically in recent years as one of the most challenging symptoms of Long COVID. Many modern medical experts agree that brain fog can be attributed to inflammation in the brain caused by "persistent immune activation after the initial infection subsides," according to the National Institutes of Health's Dr. Avindra Nath. This immune activation may be caused by lingering virus that the immune system is unable to clear, which can form biofilms resistant to immunity and pharmaceuticals, as well as virus-triggered autoimmunity and inflammation. Furthermore, gut dysbiosis, or a decrease in gut microbial diversity, often causes inflammatory diseases in various systems, and imbalances in gut microbiome are also believed to result in brain fog, according to a new study from a University of Pennsylvania research team.

While this is a common symptom seen in Long COVID, chronic Lyme disease, and Epstein-Barr, modern medical understanding of brain fog is still in its infancy, with no approved treatments and few studies done. Fortunately, this is a condition with a long history of treatment in Chinese medicine, and various healing modalities within this ancient medical system can provide invaluable tools for treating the symptoms that modern medicine has yet to provide answers for.

Chinese herbal formulas use multiple approaches to combat brain fog—the herbal constituents can break down biofilms, clear inflammation, and regulate gut flora imbalance, all of which mitigate neuroinflammation. Qigong is another well-known modality for alleviating brain fog; according to a 2021 study, qigong increases hippocampal volume, reduces markers of inflammation, and provides neurocognitive benefits that may help slow cognitive decline.

In the following sections, an extensive range of appropriate formulas widely available in

the West, as well as a single-herb recommendation, medical qigong exercises, and self-massage techniques, are discussed. But first, let's learn more about brain fog and related concepts through an historical Chinese medical lens.

An Historian's Overview of Brain Fog in Traditional Chinese Medicine

According to early medical texts, memory and clarity of mind are associated with the function of a number of critical Organs (zang 藏), particularly the Kidney, Spleen, and Heart. The conditions associated with impairments of memory and alertness, and the general difficulty in concentration and lack of focus we refer to as "brain fog," are discussed in a number of Chinese medical texts. We find a related cluster of concepts and terms in these texts, such as various forms of wang 忘 (forgetfulness) and chi 痴

(senselessness). In certain contexts, the latter term is connected with kuang 狂 (madness), but a specific form that involves diminishment of normal capacities, which has led some scholars to translate it as "dementia."

The causes of brain fog, forgetfulness, and senselessness are generally associated with dysfunctions of the Organs that become more common with increasing age, but the Chinese medical tradition also recognized cases of brain fog in younger people.

According to the Suwen section of the Huangdi Neijing, forgetfulness, along with a host of other related mental conditions, such as huo 惑 (confusion) and bei 悲 (sadness), are related to imbalances of qi and Blood in the Heart (xin 心). This can happen for a variety of reasons, ranging from seasonal effects to improper diet, suggesting a host of related psychological conditions. Interestingly, Suwen consistently links forgetfulness with sadness, with both resulting from yang qi entering the Heart improperly. The Suwen contrasts this state with that leading to excitement and anger: "When the Blood collects above and the qi collects below [in the Heart], the Heart is vexed and the patient tends to be angry. When the blood collects below and the qi collects above [in the Heart], patients behave disorderly and tend to forget."

Zhang Zhongjing's Shanghanlun (Treatise on Injuries from Cold and Miscellaneous Diseases) discusses the condition in its chapter on yang ming (陽明) disease, a disorder of qi in which heat enters the Blood. This text also ties brain fog to a host of gastrointestinal disorders, connecting both to a congealment of Blood failing to flow properly, in conjunction with heat. Certain texts attribute

the lack of concentration typical of brain fog to "distress and restlessness" (fanzao 煩躁) that can distract and cause lack of focus, in addition to a number of other symptoms. All such symptoms can additionally be connected to kuang (madness) more generally, as described in the Diankuang chapter of the Lingshu section of Huangdi Neijing.

Cases of the kind of brain fog typically seen in younger people, associated with aftereffects of viruses, exhaustion, or other similar features, is understood in the tradition as resulting from Dampness, which can be a response to heat and inflammation, and causes deficiency of qi in the Spleen. This is also linked to the digestive system, suggesting additional treatment through diet.

Many treatments are offered in the medical texts for the cluster of ailments associated with brain fog, including familiar techniques such as acupuncture, herbal remedies, and others aimed at restoring proper functioning of the related Organs and circulation of Blood and qi.

A Clinician's Approach to Brain Fog in Traditional Chinese Medicine

Brain fog is rarely an isolated symptom. It is shaping up to be a key symptom in Long COVID, and it has been associated with Epstein-Barr, Lyme disease, fibromyalgia, chronic fatigue syndrome, irritable bowel syndrome, small intestine bacterial overgrowth, and perimenopausal syndromes. One common factor among these conditions is what Chinese medicine refers to as Internal Dampness. "Dampness" is a term used in Chinese medicine to connote poor absorption and elimination, resulting in excess fluid sitting in the body, and thus, compromised digestion.

Today, we are awash in ultra-processed foods, with uneven access to alternatives. The result is not only compromised digestion but also inflammation and disruption of the microbiome. When we take into account the current medical theory that brain fog is attributed to inflammation in the brain caused by "persistent immune activation after the initial infection subsides," combined with the role that viruses and biofilms play, resulting in brain fog (especially post-infection, as is the case with Long COVID, Epstein-Barr, and chronic Lyme disease), a picture emerges that is quite consistent with the more direct insight of Chinese medicine: As a medical system that recognizes the connection between the body and the mind, as well as the emotions and spirit (shen), we are able to address many chronic disorders, such as brain fog, that are not well understood and are currently considered "untreatable" from a Western medicine perspective.

Causes of Brain Fog: Chinese Medicine Patterns

In Chinese medicine, brain fog falls into a few basic patterns. Most of these center on the Earth and Water phases and the Organ systems of the Spleen and Kidney. The Spleen can become deficient, causing poor digestion, bloating, and fatigue. When Dampness collects due to a failure of the Spleen's digestive function, feelings of heaviness and inertia arise, as well as loose stools.

There can also be dizziness, numbness, and unsteadiness. The Kidney is strongly implicated because it is the source of yang and supports all life functions at the root. The Kidney also has a very strong relationship to the Brain, and so diminished function in the realm of clarity and thought also implicates the Kidney. Feelings of cold and greater fatigue are signs of Kidney involvement. In addition, phlegm accumulation, which can either be tangible as in mucus or intangible as in the form of clouded sense perceptions, often plays a role in brain fog. Blood Deficiency, which in many cases describes inhibited circulation, can also fail to provide adequate stimulation to the brain, leading to brain fog.

Remedies for Brain Fog

Herbal Formulas for Brain Fog

Following are herbal medicines vital for phlegm and Dampness, the primary culprits of brain fog, including herbs such as Fu Ling, Bai Zhu, Ban Xia, and Ren Shen (ginseng, which is discussed as a single-herb supplement later in this chapter). These are important herbs that appear in multiple formulas in this section. Refer to chapter 3 for more information on taking herbal formulas.

Gui Ling Zhu Gan Tang 苓桂朮甘湯 (Poria, Cinnamon Twig, Atractylodes, and Licorice Decoction)

One of the ways to describe this formula is that it promotes Water metabolism. It can be thought of as ascending clear yang energy so the mind can be clear and, as the clouds part, the sun-showers appear—and maybe even a rainbow or two. See indications in the following table for symptoms you may be experiencing. This formula is safe for long-term use.

Herb	Function	Indications
Fu Ling	Percolates Dampness	Dizziness, mild cough
Gui Zhi	Warms and circulates yang qi	Palpitations, fullness in chest
Bai Zhu	Dries Dampness	Abdominal bloating, fullness, muzzy-headed feeling
Zhi Gan Cao	Harmonizes, benefits Earth	Loose stools, thirst without dryness

Bu Nao Wan 补脑丸 (Brain Repair Pill)

Bu Nao Wan is a complex and widely available formula that is safe and balanced for long-term use. It supplements energy and resources, drains Dampness that gives rise to foggy feelings and a clouded sensorium, and nourishes Blood to promote healthy circulation within the Brain. Spirit-calming herbs also help the nervous system be calmer and more still to promote feelings of centeredness and ease. Herbs that clear Internal Wind are also included to address the erratic quality of thoughts accompanying brain fog. You might consider this a general strengthening formula to promote clear thinking, concentration, and calm openness—that is, if you experience difficulty thinking clearly, have poor focus, or feel withdrawn and stuck.

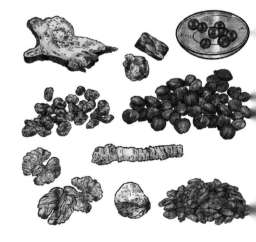

Herb	Function	Indications
Suan Zao Ren	Calms spirit (shen), eliminates deficient vexation	Easily agitated, inflammation in the nervous system
Dang Gui	Tonifies Blood	Feeling slightly cold, pale skin, dry skin and nails
Hu Tao Ren	Directly supports the Brain through tonifying yang	Cold low back, slight back pain
Rou Cong Rong	Tonifies yang	Frequent urination, cold feelings
Gou Qi Zi	Tonifies Blood	Dry eyes, fatigue, pallor
Wu Wei Zi	Astringes (gathers thoughts), calms spirit	Irritability, poor concentration
Bai Zi Ren	Nourishes Heart Blood	Insomnia, poor focus, disorganized, easily distracted
Yi Zhi Ren	Astringes the Kidney, benefits essence	Frequent urination, loose stools
Tian Ma	Extinguishes Wind	Headache (whole head feels heavy), dizziness, numbness in the extremities, tremors
Hu Po	Calms spirit (shen)	Mental agitation, insomnia
Yuan Zhi	Harmonizes Heart and Kidney	Diminished awareness, erratic thought patterns
Tian Nan Xing	Dries Dampness, disperses phlegm	Dizziness, difficult breathing or cough, numbness
Tian Zhu Huang	Clears and transforms phlegm	Difficulty finding words, tics, slight tremors
Long Gu	Settles and calms spirit	Emotional stress, agitation, insomnia

Zhen Wu Tang 真武湯 (True Warrior Decoction)

This formula's translated name speaks of the deity of the North, which is associated with Water. In addition to regulating Water metabolism, it warms with the powerful Kidney yang herb Fu Zi (aconite). Fu Zi not only warms but also consolidates and strengthens life force at its very root, and it promotes strength necessary to face life with vigor and clarity. Thus, it is like the sun driving the entire Water cycle with its life-giving rays. Use this if you experience fatigue, edema, or other symptoms listed here. *If you run hot, avoid this formula.*

Herb	Function	Indications
Fu Zi	Warms Imperial Fire	Fatigue, cold feeling, lassitude, muscle twitching
Fu Ling	Promotes urination, percolates Dampness	Edema, Water accumulation, dizziness, palpitations, instability
Bai Zhu	Leaches Dampness to build Earth	Abdominal bloating, heavy feeling, loose stools
Sheng Jiang	Warms and circulates, promoting Water metabolism	Poor appetite, loose stools
Bai Shao	Protects and nourishes Blood to ease circulation	Abdominal pain, diminished peripheral circulation

Spleen Qi Deficiency

This is a common diagnosis when treating brain fog, with signs of general fatigue and diminished function. Loose stools, abdominal bloating, diminished appetite, poor energy, and foggy-headedness can be a common presentation. The chart here compares a few common remedies that share ingredients like Bai Zhu, Fu Ling, Ren Shen, and Gan Cao. Note that the last word of each formula here and throughout the book—tang (decoction or "soup") or san (powder)—is the original, ancient dosage form, but all of these are more widely available today in wan (pill) form.

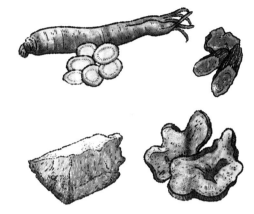

Formula Name	Medicinals Used	Indications
Si Jun Zi Tang	Ren Shen Bai Zhu Fu Ling Zhi Gan Cao	Loose stools, gastritis, bloating, fatigue
Shen Ling Bai Zhu San	Ren Shen Fu Ling Bai Zhu Shan Yao Lian Zi Rou Bian Dou Yi Yi Ren Sha Ren Jie Geng Gan Cao	Diarrhea, pale face, fatigue, weakness, abdominal distention, poor appetite
Bu Zhong Yi Qi Tang	Huang Qi Ren Shen Zhi Gan Cao Bai Zhu Chen Pi Chai Hu Sheng Ma Dang Gui	Tired body, weak limbs, low energy, shallow breathing, signs of prolapse, foggy-headedness, bruising easily, feelings of heat or slight feverishness with exhaustion

A more pernicious Dampness can also promote feelings of clouded senses. This type of Dampness may result in more bloating, fullness in the abdomen, and loose stools. Inflammation can drive the body to produce fluids that become enmeshed in a feedback loop of heat and Dampness, or cold and Dampness, that can become as difficult to separate as oil in flour. Two related formulas, widely available in many forms, are compared in the following chart.

Formula Name	Medicinals Used	Indications
Er Chen Tang	Ban Xia Chen Pi Sheng Jiang Fu Ling Wu Mei Zhi Gan Cao	Stuffy feelings in the chest and head, nausea and vomiting, dizziness, heavy extremities
Wen Dan Tang (commonly used for many psychological and neurological conditions, such as PTSD, ADHD, and anxiety)	Chen Pi Zhi Shi Ban Xia Zhu Ru Sheng Jiang Fu Ling Da Zao Gan Cao	Insomnia, vexation, palpitations, stuffy chest, easily frightened

Single-Herb Supplement for Brain Fog: Ginseng

As we learned earlier, many experts attribute brain fog to inflammation in the brain caused by immune activation that persists after an initial viral infection, as well as gut dysbiosis, which is now believed to result in brain fog, as supported by new studies. There are a few Chinese medicine herbs that may be particularly suitable as a single-herb tonic, such as ginseng, ginkgo biloba, and lion's mane. Although there seems to be increasing anecdotal evidence of ginkgo biloba's and lion's mane's abilities to improve brain fog, there is not yet extensive research on these herbs for this purpose. However, there is extensive research to support the beneficial effects of ginseng and ginsenosides (ginseng's active compounds) on the reduction of neuroinflammation. Asian (or Korean) red ginseng extracts have the ability to inhibit the activation of both NLRP3 and AIM2 inflammasome in bone marrow-derived macrophages (BMDM cells). Furthermore, multiple studies indicate that ginseng can regulate gut microbiota diversity and increase some probiotics (such as Bifidobacterium, Bacteroides, Verrucomicrobia, and Akkermansia), as well as reduce pathogenic bacteria (such as Deferribacteres, Lactobacillus, and Helicobacter) against various diseases.

While Chinese medicinal herbs are rarely taken on their own, ginseng is usually regarded as a safe single-herb health elixir for short- or medium-term use, and it can be helpful for reducing brain fog, improving memory, and boosting cognitive function. One of the most widely used herbs in the world, ginseng also happens to be one of the most studied—one report from 2018 counted more than 3,400 published research papers on the herb since the 1980s!

Ginseng is typically used in Chinese medicine as a tonic for weak or exhausted bodies and for anyone who is convalescing. It's often recommended for people experiencing lack of concentration, memory loss, or brain fog, and its restorative, cognition-enhancing properties have made it popular as a supplement for post-COVID brain fog. Asian families often add it to hearty tonic soups for people recovering from illness or who have weaker constitutions—my mom often adds it to chicken soups, simmered in a clay pot over the course of several hours.

Ginseng Varieties

There are many varieties of ginseng, the two most relevant being Asian (Korean) ginseng and American ginseng. Furthermore, there are two common types of ginseng preparation: white and red. White ginseng has simply been dried, whereas red ginseng has further been steamed. The difference in processing results in different therapeutic applications. One study concluded that both red and white ginseng preparations have a strong effect on brain activity but their modes of action on the brain are different. Unfortunately, many researchers, especially outside of East Asia, are unaware of these differences and don't distinguish between the two in their research trials.

A randomized, double-blind, placebo-controlled trial determined that taking Asian ginseng for six months has a positive effect on cognitive improvement, particularly on visual memory function in Korean subjects with mild cognitive impairment. This study also noted that its results strongly supported the results from two previous studies, which also demonstrated the positive effect of ginseng on cognitive function, and added that there were no related adverse side effects. The conclusion was that ginseng has cognition-enhancing effects and can be used safely. Similarly, a randomized, double-blind, placebo-controlled, crossover study from an Australian research team evaluating American ginseng's effects on cognitive function concluded there was robust working memory enhancement following the administration of American ginseng. Ginseng can be combined with ginkgo biloba, an herb that may be beneficial in the treatment of cognitive disorders.

Ginseng Decoction for Brain Fog

In Chinese medicinal cuisine, ginseng is often consumed as a "tea," or as an herb added to meat soups. While the verdict is still out on whether Asian (Korean) or American ginseng is the better choice for brain fog, in TCM terms, American ginseng is considered cooling whereas Asian ginseng is considered warming. Those who have poor circulation, are frequently cold, and/or have digestive issues may be better suited to Asian ginseng, whereas those with more "heat-y" constitutions and who have excessive thirst or dry mouth, irritability, and reddish complexions may be better suited to American ginseng. *Ginseng may not be for you if you experience insomnia or nervousness after taking it.*

Ginseng Concoction for Brain Fog

Yield: Makes 3 to 4 cups (720 to 960 ml)

- **3 to 9 g dried ginseng root**

- **3 to 4 cups (720 to 960 ml) water**

- **Honey, to sweeten (optional)**

  In a small pot over medium heat, combine the ginseng and water. Bring to a boil, then decrease the heat to low and simmer for about an hour. If using sliced ginseng, simmer for a shorter time—30 minutes is adequate. Strain and add honey to taste.

Medical Qigong for Brain Fog

In general, brain fog is a symptom of lack of Blood and qi flow upward toward the head. Potentially, this can be due to impeded Heart-Lung and/or digestive function, leading to a stagnation of qi, Blood, and body fluids throughout the body, in particular toward the head. As previously discussed, these are all conditions that can potentially occur after contracting viral infections, and brain fog is a common symptom of Long COVID—fortunately, one that can be addressed by Chinese medicine and qigong. The following sequence of exercises has been designed specifically to address this set of symptoms. As there may be several distinct physiological causes of this brain fog, this set of qigong exercises is designed to be practiced as a sequence in this order to address multiple potential causes. Keep the following general guidelines in mind as you complete the practice.

General Rules of Qigong Practice

- Wear comfortable, loose-fitting clothes and shoes.

- Keep your eyes half-closed and maintain a soft gaze.

- Keep your tongue gently touching the roof of your mouth.

- Breath gently using long, slow, deep, quiet breaths, in and out of the nose. If you can hear yourself breathing, you are probably breathing too loudly.

- Do not train with a full stomach. It is best to wait two hours after eating before training.

- Do not train in a thunderstorm or outdoors in a foggy or smoky environment. It is best to find a tidy place with a good circulation of fresh air, indoors or outdoors, to train in.

- Those who are pregnant or menstruating are advised to abstain from unsupervised practice.

**Exercise 1: Kai He 開合
(Opening and Closing)**

This exercise opens the fascial tissue around the chest cavity, creating space around the Lung and Heart, allowing for improved functioning of these Organs and ease of diaphragmatic movement. In Chinese medical theory, these Organs are incredibly important because they control the Blood and qi of the entire body. They are also Organs often targeted by COVID. Furthermore, the Heart is said to be the emperor of the body. In addition, this exercise helps open the shoulder joints, which if tight can pull on the neck fascia, in turn impeding Blood, qi, and fluid flow to the head, which is a possible factor in brain fog.

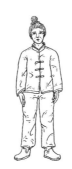
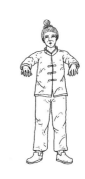

1. Stand naturally, feet facing forward, arms by your sides, breathing evenly.

2. Breathe in and raise your arms directly to the front, palms facing down.

3. Continuing to breathe in, bring your arms into a trident shape and expand the body with breath from the toes to the fingers.

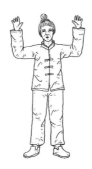
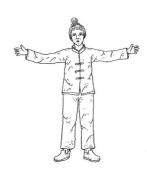

4. Begin to exhale, dropping your arms into a rough T shape, with the palms facing forward.

5. Continue to exhale while contracting the body and bringing the palms together slowly at about shoulder height. Try to feel a growing sense of pressure between the palms as they get closer together.

6. Continue to breathe out, drawing the breath down the body through the feet into the ground as your arms drop to the sides of the body.

7. Repeat this exercise 9 to 36 times.

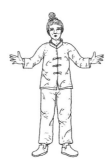
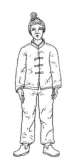

Exercise 2: Shaking 搖

Shaking is a common practice in the Chinese healing arts. Its function is to unblock the meridians of the entire body and facilitate the vertical free flow of qi. In affecting the Heart and Lung, COVID can affect Blood and qi flow throughout the body. It can also result in stagnation of body fluids, leading to Dampness in the body's meridians.

1. Stand naturally, feet facing forward, arms by your sides, breathing evenly.

2. Vibrate and shake your entire body, wrists, ankles, and heels in particular, for 2 to 10 minutes (you can shake longer, depending on your state of health or physical ability). The shaking should not be a jiggle, up and down. Instead, place more emphasis on the downward motion, as if you're shaking a large sack of rice and the bulk of weight collects toward the bottom.

3. Attention can be focused on areas of the body that exhibit significant tension or tightness.

4. Stand still afterward for a similar length of time.

Self-Massage for Brain Fog

Rubbing Belly

This exercise will assist in the healthy functioning of the digestive system, which, if disrupted, can be a major factor contributing to brain fog. You can perform this abdomen massage more or less, depending on how much digestive factors and internal Dampness are contributing to your brain fog. You may benefit from the higher repetitions if you're experiencing poor digestion and signs of internal Dampness, such as bloating, water retention, or loose stools.

1. Place the palm of one hand on the back of the other hand.

2. Breathe in fully and, on the exhale, use both hands, one on top of the other, to massage firmly down the midline of the abdomen to the pubic bone. Repeat 36 to 108 times.

3. Place both hands on the lower abdomen under the belly button. Massage slow, counterclockwise circles around the belly button, gradually increasing the size of the circles. Repeat 36 to 108 times.

4. Massage slow, clockwise circles around the belly button, gradually decreasing the size of the circles. Repeat 36 to 108 times.

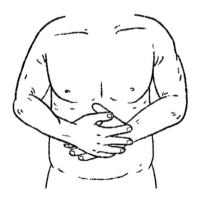

Head Massage

This exercise is designed to bring blood and qi flow back to the head and is usually performed after poor blood/qi flow has been identified as the underlying cause of brain fog. It can also be performed at the onset of symptoms, but its efficacy may depend on the degree to which underlying causes have been dealt with.

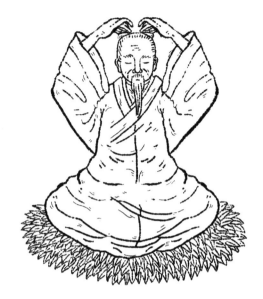

1. Comb the fingers through the hair and across the scalp.

2. Tap firmly with the fingertips on the scalp, back of the head, face, and jaw, focusing on any areas of tension.

3. Alternate between tapping and combing for 5 to 10 minutes, or until a sensation of warmth and/or flow arises in the head.

Conclusion

If you are suffering from brain fog caused by illness that has left you fatigued and weak, you may benefit from reading chapter 5, Depression, which touches upon these concepts.

Next, we will explore the Chinese medicine approach to trauma.

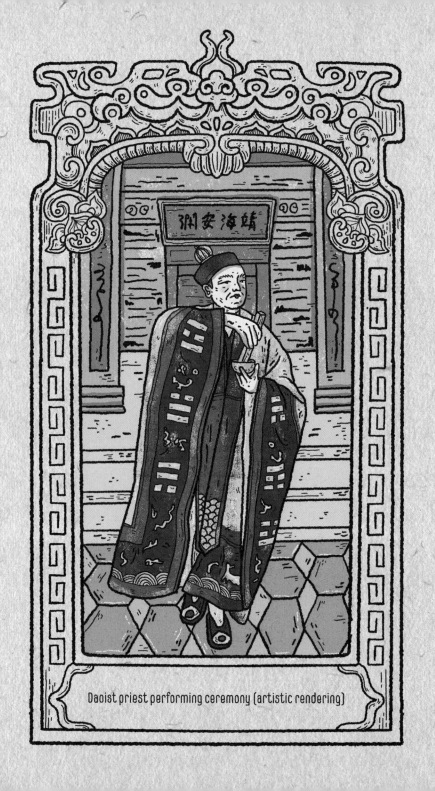

Daoist priest performing ceremony (artistic rendering)

CHAPTER 9

TRAUMA

There are a remarkable number of resources in Chinese medicine for trauma relief, primarily focused on rebalancing and restoration. Unlike other mental health conditions, trauma is the subject of a relatively large body of modern Chinese medical literature in the West, representing both protocols aimed at clinicians and philosophical approaches aimed at trauma sufferers. Those who are familiar with psychology's approach to coping strategies for traumatic stress reactions may be surprised to learn how much is similar to a classical Chinese or Daoist philosophical approach. For this reason, continuing to learn more about Daoist philosophy, such as from philosophers like Zhuangzi, may benefit trauma sufferers.

Trauma is a complex condition, involving aspects of many other emotional, psychological, and physiological conditions. What makes an experience traumatic? Here are some defining characteristics:

1. Overwhelms the nervous system

2. Violates boundaries

3. Disrupts relationality

4. Severs connections

5. Admits feelings of powerlessness

6. Damages the sense of meaning

7. Inhibits the sense of self

8. Disrupts contact with the self

9. Instigates or stimulates collapse/separation of yin and yang

Responses to these circumstances are outlined in the definitions of post-traumatic stress disorder (PTSD) and complex PTSD as specific symptoms, and are also increasingly understood to play roles in some personality disorders. All of this is to suggest that, as a system, there is an aspect of our anatomy and physiology, according to Chinese medicine, that resonates with this deep, enduring, and profound aspect of our being so that experience becomes amenable to influence, change, and healing.

After enduring a traumatic experience, a person's qi is said to be "scattered," leaving you with a sense of being disconnected from your body or self. There are many tools in the Chinese medicine toolbox that may overlap with a modern Western approach, including psychotherapy—what were called "talking cures" in ancient China and known to be practiced by Zhu Danxi (1282–1358)—but the herbal formulas are distinct from the Western medicating approach, which focuses on sedating the mind or altering serotonin levels. The herbal approach restores one's Heart, Blood circulation, and qi to bring the body back to homeostasis. Acupuncture or acupressure can further instill a sense of self-awareness, reduce stress, and leave us with a feeling of ease instead of fright, shock, or numbness.

Although the following suggestions are made by a licensed practitioner with significant experience with mental health disorders, those who suffer from trauma are particularly encouraged to seek professional help and guidance, and acupuncture for trauma relief is widely available in many cities and provided by nonprofits at very low or sliding scale rates.

An Historian's Overview of Trauma in Traditional Chinese Medicine

Trauma is a complicated phenomenon in the history of Chinese medicine, as it has a connection to a number of other states and conditions, both physical and mental. A number of emotions and disorders are associated with trauma, such as fear, anger, grief, and various types of anxiety and depression. According to early medical texts, excessive or extreme emotional states can bring about mental illness. Fear, anger, anxiety, fright, and sadness can have a detrimental effect on the operation of the Organs and the circulation of Blood and qi.

The Suwen section of the *Huangdi Neijing* discusses the idea of trauma, connecting it to fear, anger, and fatigue. According to the text, the Blood and qi are altered by these states in ways that lead to physical effects, such as reduction of energy and continued mental effects . . . The text reads, "Whenever a person is frightened, fearful, angry, or overworked, whether one is active or quiet, this all causes changes."

Because the movement of Blood is adversely affected by such emotional and physical shock, this creates deficiencies in various Organs, which result in related physical and psychological ailments. In particular, the Su-

wen discusses physical symptoms such as racing breath (a sign of agitation) and numbness, also claiming that features of a person's character will, in part, determine the severity of symptoms, with more sensitive people being more severely affected.

Zhang Zhongjing's *Shanghanlun* also associates trauma with such physical effects as sweating and heart palpitations. Such physical manifestations in the absence of a direct precipitating cause can demonstrate underlying emotional trauma. This demonstrates the variety of effects trauma can have on a person, as well as its complexity. Different Organs are sources of particular emotions that can lead to and be caused by trauma. For example, the Liver is associated with fright and shock.

Severe and unaddressed trauma can have negative effects that can even undermine one's ability to perform basic life necessities by negatively affecting one's Jing 精 (essence). The *Shanghanlun* considers a kind of fright that rises to the level of "madness"—jingkuang 惊狂—attributing it to the collapse of yang in the Heart. "Madness" here refers to a kind of manic state in which actions are heightened and frantic. Traumatic fright is also associated with jingxian 惊癇, which is a kind of opposite to jingkuang, in which trauma leads not to manic action but instead to withdrawal and silence.

Given trauma's complexity, treatment is also varied in the medical tradition. Individual symptoms such as palpitations, sweating, nervousness, or the variety of other physical and mental symptoms that result from trauma can all be treated. A more direct solution to the causes of trauma, however, involves the restoration of proper circulation of Blood and qi from the Heart. This treatment can involve methods such as ingesting herbs, acupuncture, and other physical techniques, but can also involve the encouragement and cultivation of emotions and attitudes that have the ability to counteract the problematic emotions created by trauma. The *Huangdi Neijing* presents a view of emotions in which certain emotions are able to overcome others—joy, for example, overcomes fear. For this reason, part of a treatment for trauma-based fear may be the encouragement of activities that generate joy. The seventh-century CE commentator Yang Shangshan explained, "When someone hears something enjoyable, his body and his heart will be full of delight. . . . In the case of joy, the entire body is relaxed."

A Clinician's Approach to Trauma in Traditional Chinese Medicine

The saying that all disease comes from the Heart can be understood as a testament to the role of circulation in the body. It is, of course, noteworthy that the steady, rhythmic beat of the Heart attends life. Suwen, chapter 8, describes the Heart as the emperor, and its health is of paramount importance.

One concept from the work of Dr. Leon Hammer, and from his teacher Dr. John Shen, is also attested to in Suwen, chapter 39, "Discourse on Pain." One of the most important passages regarding emotions in the entire text appears in this chapter, where a number of passages describe emotions, such as sadness and fear, creating a state in which the Upper Jiao, including the Chest, Heart, and Lung, becomes impassable. In Dr. Shen's terms, this was called Heart Closed. Zhang Zhongjing, in the *Jin Gui Yao Lue (Essential Prescriptions of the Golden Cabinet)*, describes a similar state called Xiong Bi, or Stuck Qi in the Chest. Suwen, chapter 39, also describes the influence of fright, which leaves the spirit (shen) with nowhere to settle, and produces a state of chaos in the system. Such chaos can be likened to a loss of contact between yin and yang—a vulnerable condition that affects the circulation, access to internal resources, and resilience to handling stressful stimuli. The effect of all of these patterns can manifest almost anywhere in the body, and in any number of mental, emotional, and physical symptoms that are characterized by dysregulation.

One of the primary expressions of rhythm and movement in the body is the regular beat of the Heart, the rhythmic pulsing of the blood vessels, and the overall circulation of both Blood and nervous system impulses. Understood as a process, yin and yang describe these movements as expansion and contraction occurring throughout the entire body system. Depending on where there are vulnerabilities in different tissues and Organs, the homeostatic effects of healthy Blood circulation and nervous system tone will be affected. For example, an arrested rhythm in the vasculature of the head is associated with migraines whereas impaired microcirculation in the gut can be associated with irritable bowel syndrome. Within the nervous system, we can recognize sympathetic hyperarousal as an analogous pattern. Once we begin to see these physiological processes as yin-yang alterations of circulation, then we can see just how vital the role of the Heart is in the entire body, just as the classical texts suggest. We also see how the body and mind are truly unified.

Thus, the clinical approach to working with trauma involves this precise dynamic. At one level, focusing on the circulation and promoting its movement is the most important factor. But there is a dimension of the Blood that conventional medicine cannot quantify, and that is the role of the spirit and awareness as it is housed in the Heart Organ system and circulated via the Blood. In Chinese medicine, circulation is not merely a closed circuit but a spiral opening to the cosmos—a conduit for the healing force of the infinitely creative expression of the whole. When we promote the health of the Heart, we invite this expression to refashion any experience we have ever had—even traumatic ones.

Then, we can view the diagnostic criteria of Western psychology in a new light as well as understanding the importance of somatic psychology approaches that have become well known. As an MD and psychiatrist as well as a Chinese medicine practitioner, Dr. Leon Hammer was involved with some of the somatic methods, but for him, Chinese medicine was the most powerful and comprehensive approach he found to treat trauma.

Remedies for Trauma

Traditional Chinese herbal patent (standardized) medicines are generally safe to use, and this book features formulas regarded as well-balanced. Look for the symptoms that match your experience, paying special attention to physical symptoms in this section. In the experience of clinicians such as Brandt Stickley, the following herbal formulas are acceptable to take even if you are currently on other medication, including prescription antidepressants and anxiolytics (as previously mentioned, space these out an hour from when you take herbal medication). Refer to chapter 3, which provides more detail on how to take herbal formulas. You can also seek professional help from a Chinese medicine practitioner with training in herbal medicine if you want to go further with your journey in TCM. These formulas are safe for long-term use, except Yunnan Baiyao (page 142), which is a limited protocol. Each formula can be taken for four to six weeks at full dosage, after which you can lower the dosage or take it as needed.

Herbal Formulas for Trauma

In the Shen-Hammer pulse lineage, or school of thought, the combination of Sheng Mai San (page 141) and Yunnan Baiyao (page 142) has been used to address the pattern of Heart Shock, a term for traumatic experience. Another significant contribution of the Shen-Hammer pulse tradition is the identification of pulse qualities, such as flat and inflated pulses that describe conditions when the qi and Blood in the chest cannot enter or exit and are thus stuck. This is described as a block to treatment—a state that inhibits other interventions if not addressed. "Block" is another translation of the term "bi" 閉 that occurs in the context of Xiong Bi or Chest Bi.

The Heart is impacted directly by trauma, and from its position of sovereignty in the body, this has global effects. The top three recommended formulas all correspond to restoring this Organ system using herbs that help strengthen the Heart and circulation. However, because trauma is a very complex condition, it can manifest differently throughout the body—via the head, musculature, nervous system, digestive system, and urogenital system. I have listed these by symptom at the end of page 148.

Sheng Mai San 生脈散 (Generate the Pulse Powder)

This formula regulates the pulse rhythm and rate. It comprises three herbs. Using this formula to treat trauma is unique to the Shen-Hammer lineage, but its function to regulate the rhythm is key to understanding its potential. This is a good formula if you experience racing heart rate, arrythmia, or palpitations. It should be taken until your pulse rate normalizes and becomes neither too fast nor too slow; it is also safe for longer-term use.

Herb	Function	Indications
Ren Shen Ginseng or Xi Yang Shen (American ginseng)	Tonify qi and yin fluids	Weak pulse, fatigue, weak voice
Mai Men Dong	Nourish Lung, moisten	Arrythmia, palpitations
Wu Wei Zi	Astringe and regulate Lung	Racing or irregular heart rate, anxiety

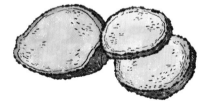

Yunnan Baiyao 云南白药 (brand name)

This proprietary medicine has a storied and enigmatic history. It is commonly recognized as a treatment for physical trauma and injury, even gunshot wounds or auto accidents, and was a staple in the emergency kit of Viet Cong soldiers. However, in the Shen-Hammer lineage, it has been used even for remote experiences of physical or emotional trauma, such as birth trauma or adverse experiences in life that occurred decades earlier. Although widely available, there is some uncertainty about its ingredients due to its proprietary nature and closely guarded recipe by its manufacturer. A quick online search, however, provides a list of major constituents, including San Qi (Panax notoginseng).

While the following provides a model for using this remedy, there is also an alternative that similarly addresses a pattern of qi and Blood Stagnation in the Heart. These capsules should always be taken with food. The course of treatment is one or two capsules twice per day for the total duration of sixty-four capsules. The powder form can also be used—look for the version that comes with a small spoon; one spoonful is equivalent to one capsule. *Avoid this formula, or seek professional guidance, if you are on blood thinners.*

1. Before bed the night before starting the protocol, take the small red pill. This is an extra-strength dose included inside every pack of Yunnan Baiyao capsules, or inside each bottle of powder. In the bottle, it is located under the cap.

2. The next day, take 1 capsule twice per day.

3. The following day, take 1 capsule 3 times per day.

4. Then, take 1 capsule 4 times per day.

5. From here, jump to the maximum of 2 capsules 4 times per day until you complete the course.

Herb	Yunnan Baiyao (capsules)

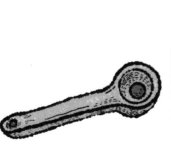
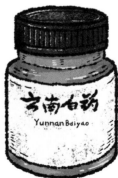

Xue Fu Zhu Yu Tang 血府逐瘀湯 (Blood Stasis Relief)

This is an alternative treatment to Yunnan Baiyao that also strongly moves qi and Blood in the Heart. This formula is also recognized as a remedy for recalcitrant insomnia and sleep disturbances as well as nightmares—all common symptoms of traumatic experience. This is a good formula if you are experiencing chest pain or heart pain, emotional or physical, or other symptoms listed here.

Herb	Function	Indications
Tao Ren Hong Hua Dang Gui Chi Shao Sheng Di Chuan Xiong	Tonify and move Blood	Fixed pain, stabbing or sharp pains, chest pain, palpitations, nightmares, labile emotions
Chai Hu Zhi Ke Gan Cao	Regulate ascending qi and descending qi to strongly move and circulate qi	Cold hands and feet, diminished circulation, pain and discomfort in ribcage
Jie Geng	Open the Lung, descend qi to disperse stagnant qi in chest	Shallow or inhibited breathing
Niu Xi	Move Blood downward to dispel stasis in chest	Body and joint pain

Herbal Formulas for Other Symptoms of Trauma

As mentioned, many of the symptoms associated with traumatic experience can be understood through the traditional concept of fright, and even kuang. However, some patterns of Blood stasis, especially in the chest and pelvis, can be related to trauma. Menstrual pain and irregularity can also be associated with the inhibition of circulation as discussed. The chart on the opposite page highlights some specific relevant formulas to treat trauma, some more common than others, that include other key indications. You can further identify the most relevant formula for you depending on other symptoms you may be experiencing.

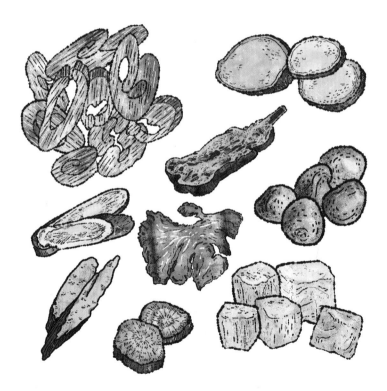

Herbal Formula	Indications
Dang Gui Shao Yao San	Abdominal and menstrual pain
Dang Gui Si Ni Tang	Cold hands and feet, sciatica, diminished circulation (a major boost to Blood circulation)
Tao He Cheng Qi Tang	Fixed, stabbing pain in the abdomen, extreme emotion
Suan Zao Ren Tang	Insomnia, anxiety
An Shen Ding Zhi Wan	Insomnia, anxiety, palpitations
Wen Dan Tang	Fearfulness, insomnia
Gan Mai Da Zao Tang	Weeping, sadness, grief
Ben Tun Tang	Neck pain, buzzing sensations, anxiety, nausea, or epigastric pain
Xiao Yao San or Jia Wei Xiao Yao San	Irritability, depression, stress, loose stools, irregular menstruation

Acupressure for Trauma

Many suggestions for working with traumatic experience mirror those for anxiety (see chapter 6). Thus, any practice that brings awareness into the body and establishes a sense of safety and internal stillness will be beneficial. This could be as simple as cupping your hands on your shoulders, or applying gentle pressure with both hands to your abdomen simply to experience your own presence and touch, and breathing into the area and acknowledging that this is your own experience and your own body. However, alongside this type of self-care, a few points are specifically indicated. Perform the acupressure for a few minutes or as long as it feels comfortable.

PC 6 Nei Guan 内关 (Inner Gate)

This exercise is good any time there is an oppressive sensation in the chest, a disruption of heart rhythm, or nausea. Just a few finger-widths above the wrist crease, on the inside of the wrist and between the two prominent tendons, is the point known as Inner Gate. In acupuncture, this is the most important point, in Brandt Stickley's experience, for working with Stuck Qi in the Chest that is often a sign of trauma. He uses a needling technique called Leading the Qi (Dao Qi) to promote a sensation that travels up the arm and into the chest. Patients often feel an opening sensation and warmth, both of which are liberating. With self-acupressure, harnessing your own awareness alongside pressure at the wrist point can create a kind of circuit that produces similar results. It may feel subtle, or you may feel as if you are just imagining it, but this can still be beneficial.

TB 5 Wai Guan 外关 (Outer Gate)

Exactly opposite PC 6 Nei Guan, on the outside of the wrist, is another acupoint—TB 5 Wai Guan, meaning Outer Gate. It can even be pressed simultaneously with its counterpart, Inner Gate. This procedure aims to foster a sense of ease between the inner and outer aspects of our experience. Simple pressure with a circular motion is appropriate here to ease agitation, irritability, and overwhelm.

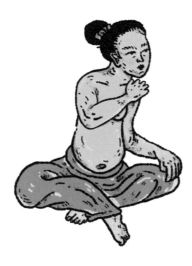

LU 1 Zhong Fu中府 (Central Residence)

Another point, LU 1 Zhong Fu, is in front of the shoulder and below the end of the collarbone, located in the first intercostal space between the first and second ribs. It will often feel sensitive, which can help identify it. Crossing the hands to contact the point on both sides is another significant way to promote openness in the chest. Additionally, this speaks to the saying that the lungs face the 100 Vessels—a way to describe an impact on the overall circulation of qi in the body. LU 1 is the first point on the channel and represents the first step toward the whole system of the acupuncture channels. It will help you experience full breath and a feeling of ease.

Acupuncture for Trauma

Acupuncture is known to work extremely well for trauma and is a particularly beneficial therapy to incorporate alongside herbal medicine. In this section, you'll learn about a popular acupuncture protocol for trauma. You can seek an acupuncturist who may needle these or other points for you, or try these points at home via acupressure or moxibustion. In the case of moxibustion, do each point for a few minutes, or until the warmth becomes uncomfortable (see page 38 for more on moxibustion). If you are already being treated weekly by an acupuncturist, you can perform this protocol between sessions for additional relief.

As seen in other sections of this text, the impact of traumatic experience is not limited to a single Organ system. Research indicates that early adverse experiences have demonstrable effects on behavior, chronic disease, and mortality. In Chinese medicine, there is a system of acupuncture channels that are expressions of influences on the body that unfold alongside the lifelong processes of birth, growth, maturation, decline, and death. These channels are called the Eight Extraordinary Channels, and they are particularly relevant to working with the aftermath of trauma.

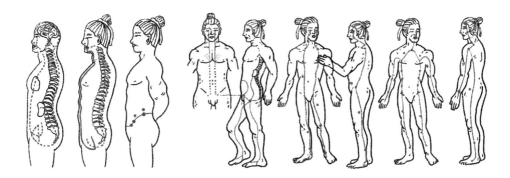

Eight Extraordinary Channels

There are many approaches to the Eight Extraordinary Channels from within different traditions and texts. Here is one simple model you can also work with through acupressure or moxibustion, based on descriptions from the first-century medical text, *Nan Jing*.

Channel and Master Point	Function	Symptoms, Patterns
1. Du SI 3	Sea of Yang Qi, govern yang	Stiffness of spine, seizures, spasm, mental agitation, autonomy
2. Ren LU 7	Sea of Yin Qi, govern yin	Internal and abdominal pain and obstruction, bonding, connection to resources
3. Chong SP 4	Sea of Blood, Sea of Channels	Counterflow, inhibition of full circulation, deep communication of spirit throughout the whole body
4. Dai GB 41	Bind channels, govern ascending and descending qi	Cold and pain in lower back and abdomen, weakness of legs, suppression of feeling
5. Yinwei PC 6	Connect and coordinate yin channels; interior	Heart pain, annoyance, loss of will, loss of self-control, identifying and connecting to resources, self-sufficiency
6. Yangwei TB 5	Connect and coordinate yang channels; exterior	Suffering from heat and cold, difficulties from external insults and internal reactions
7. Yinqiao KI 6	Regulate movement of yin, laterality, inner tension of lower extremities, brain and eyes, and sleep/waking	Inner tension, pain that is hard to identify, inner narratives about experience, somnolence
8. Yangqiao UB 62	Regulate movement of yang, laterality, outer tension of lower extremities, regulate brain and eyes, sleep/waking	Outer tension, generalized pain, insomnia

Chong and Yinwei comprise a pair—SP 4 and PC 6. Over the years, many patients have shared that treatments on the Chong Mai have been the most powerful they have experienced. According to Brandt Stickley, this is because the Chong Mai represents an interface between what has been and what is possible. Being fully ourselves often requires a willingness to dare and this means being fully present and embodying what the Chong represents. Combined with the point Yinwei PC 6, which is identified in the *Nan Jing* as addressing Heart Pain, the inner turn that allows you to connect to a sense of resources and strength can be established as a felt-sense.

The Eight Extraordinary Channels have a long history of association with meditation and inner work, and we can access this easily by simply focusing and contemplating on how we feel the vigorous and resourced flow of vitality within us, mediated by the free and powerful flow of circulation. Another approach is to work with the master point of each meridian and contemplate its function using the method just described.

Conclusion

Since these chapters are organized by Western terminology, if you are suffering from trauma, you may also want to explore chapter 4, Insomnia; chapter 5, Depression; and chapter 6, Anxiety, which may have significant overlap with trauma in terms of approach and treatment, especially anxiety.

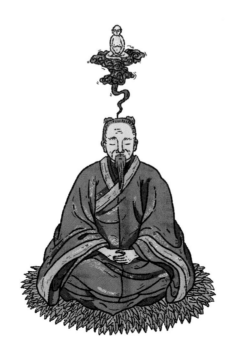

References

Introduction

Liu, William Guangling. (2015). *The Chinese Market Economy 1000–1500*. State University of New York Press.

Chaffee, John W. (2015). *The Cambridge History of China Volume 5 Part Two Sung China, 960–1279*. Cambridge University Press

Unschuld, Paul. (1984). *Medicine in China: A History of Ideas*. University of California Press.

Maciocia, Giovanni. (2015). *The Foundations of Chinese Medicine: A Comprehensive Text* (3rd ed.). Churchill Livingstone.

Chapter 1

Unschuld, Paul. (1984). *Medicine in China: A History of Ideas*. University of California Press.

Chapter 3

Cheng, Y.C. (2011, October). "Why and How to Globalize Traditional Chinese Medicine," *Journal of Traditional and Complement Medicine*, 1(1), 1-4. doi: 10.1016/s2225-4110(16)30050-5.

Petric, Z., Žuntar, I., Putnik, P., and Bursać Kovačević, D. (2020, December). "Food-Drug Interactions with Fruit Juices," *Foods*, 10(1), 33. doi: 10.3390/foods10010033.

Belayneh, A., and Molla F. (2020, July). "The Effect of Coffee on Pharmacokinetic Properties of Drugs: A Review," *BioMed Research International*. doi: 10.1155/2020/7909703.

Jia, W., Gao, W.Y., Yan, Y.Q., Wang, J., Xu, Z.H., Zheng, W.J., and Xiao, P.G. (2004, August). "The rediscovery of ancient Chinese herbal formulas." *Phytotherapy Research*, 18(8), 681-686. doi: 10.1002/ptr.1506.

Zhou, X, Seto, S.W., Chang, D., Kiat, H., Razmovski-Naumovski, V., Chan, K., and Bensoussan, A. (2016, July). "Synergistic Effects of Chinese Herbal Medicine: A Comprehensive Review of Methodology and Current Research." *Frontiers in Pharmacology*, 7, 201. doi: 10.3389/fphar.2016.00201.

Zhang, A., Sun, H., and Wang, X. (2014, April). "Potentiating Therapeutic Effects by Enhancing Synergism Based on Active Constituents from Traditional Medicine." *Phytotherapy Research*, 28(4), 526-533. doi: 10.1002/ptr.5032.

Zhang, Z., Schiffers, P., Jansen, G., Vrolijk, M., Vangireken, P., and Haenen, G. (2018, February). "The Cardiovascular Side Effects of Ma Huang Due to Its Use in Isolation in the Western World," *European Journal of Integrative Medicine*, 18, 18-22. www.sciencedirect.com/science/article/pii/S1876382018300155?via%3Dihub

Agrawal, S., and Khazaeni, B. (2024, January). "Acetaminophen Toxicity." Treasure Island, FL: *StatPearls Publishing*. www.ncbi.nlm.nih.gov/books/NBK441917/

Potash, Shana. (2015, September-October). "Arsenic Added to Cancer Therapy After Studies in China." *NIH Global Health Matters Newsletter*, 15(5). www.fic.nih.gov/News/GlobalHealthMatters/september-october-2015/Pages/china-arsenic-cancer-therapy.aspx

Rao, Y., Li, R., and Zhang, D. (2013). "A Drug from Poison: How the Therapeutic Effect of Arsenic Trioxide on Acute Promyelocytic Leukemia Was Discovered," *Science China Life Sciences*, 56, 495-502. https://doi.org/10.1007/s11427-013-4487-z

Yan, B., Zhu, S., Wang, Y., Da, G., and Tian, G. (2020, June). "Effect of Acupuncture on Chronic Pain with Depression: A Systematic Review," *Evidence-Based Complementary and Alternative Medicine*, 7479459. doi: 10.1155/2020/7479459.

Li, Bing. (2015). "Defining Music Therapy: Integrating the Chinese Perspective and the United States-Influenced Model of Music Therapy" [Unpublished master's thesis]. https://core.ac.uk/download/213413708.pdf

Hugenholtz, J. (2013). "Traditional Biotechnology for New Foods and Beverages," *Current Opinion in Biotechology*, 24, 155-159.

Hidaka, B.H. (2012). "Depression as a Disease of Modernity: Explanations for Increasing Prevalence," *Journal of Affective Disorders*, 140, 205-214. doi: 10.1016/j.jad.2011.12.036.

Colla, J., Buka, S., Harrington, D., and Murphy, J.M. (2006). "Depression and Modernization: A Cross-Cultural Study of Women," *Social Psychiatry and Psychiatric Epidemiology*, 41, 271-279. doi: 10.1007/s00127-006-0032-8.

Sugimoto, K., Takeuchi, H., Nakagawa, K., and Matsuoka, Y. (2018, October 8). "Hyperthermic Effect of Ginger (*Zingiber officinale*) Extract-Containing Beverage on Peripheral Skin Surface Temperature in Women," *Evidence-Based Complementary and Alternative Medicine*, 3207623. doi: 10.1155/2018/3207623.

Knez, E., Kadac-Czapska, K., and Grembecka, M. (2023). "Effect of Fermentation on the Nutritional Quality of the Selected Vegetables and Legumes and Their Health Effects," *Life*, 13(3), 655. https://doi.org/10.3390/life13030655

Ba, D.M., Gao, X., Al-Shaar, L., Muscat, J.E., Chinchilli, V.M., Beelman, R.B., and Richie, J.P. (2021, November 1). "Mushroom Intake and Depression: A Population-Based Study Using Data from the US National Health and Nutrition Examination Survey (NHANES), 2005-2016." *Journal of Affective Disorders*, 294, 686-692. doi: 10.1016/j.jad.2021.07.080.

Chapter 4

Gilbert, S.S., van den Heuvel, C.J., Ferguson, S.A., and Dawson, D. (2004, April). "Thermoregulation as a Sleep Signalling System," *Sleep Medine Reviews*, 8(2), 81-93. doi: 10.1016/S1087-0792(03)00023-6.

Zhang, T., Long, Y., Ma, S., and He, J. (2017, February 8). "Human Biological Rhythm in Traditional Chinese Medicine," *Journal of Traditional Chinese Medical Sciences*, 3(4). doi: 10.1016/j.jtcms.2016.12.004.

Hu, L.L., Zhang, X., Liu, W.J., Li, M., and Zhang, Y.H. (2015). "Suan Zao Ren Tang in Combination with Zhi Zi Chi Tang as a Treatment Protocol for Insomniacs with Anxiety: A Randomized Parallel-Controlled Trial," *Evidence-Based Complementary and Alternative Medicine*, 913252. doi: 10.1155/2015/913252.

Zhao, J., Wang, F., Ou, D., Zhou, B., Li, Y., Wang, H., and Deng, Q. (2023, January). "Thermoregulatory Analysis of Warm Footbaths Before Bedtime: Implications for Enhancing Sleep Quality," *Building and Environment*. doi: 10.1016/j.buildenv.2022.109788

Cao, M., Deng, Ff., Yuan, Q., et al. (2018, September 20). "Tuina for Primary Insomnia: A Meta-Analysis," *Journal of Acupuncture and Tuina Science*, 16, 236-242. doi: 10.1007/s11726-018-1056-9

Wang, X., Yin, X., Liu, P., Wang, A., Mu, W., Xu, J., Lu, W., Chen, Z., Zhou, Y., Xu, S., and Wang, Y. (2023, August 7). "The Effect of Baduanjin Qigong Combined with Five-Elements Music on Anxiety and Quality of Sleep in Asymptomatic Patients with COVID-19 infection: A Randomised Controlled Trial," *Heliyon*, 9, e18962. doi: 10.1016/j.heliyon.2023.e18962.

Chapter 5

Stone, M.B., Yaseen, Z.S., Miller, B.J., Richardville, K., Kalaria, S., and Kirsch, I. (2022). "Response to Acute Monotherapy for Major Depressive Disorder in Randomized, Placebo Controlled Trials Submitted to the US Food and Drug Administration: Individual Participant Data Analysis," *BMJ*, 378. doi: 10.1136/bmj-2021-067606.

Su, R., Fan, J., Li, T., Cao, X., Zhou, J., Han, Z., and Ma, Y. (2019, June). "Jiawei Xiaoyao Capsule Treatment for Mild to Moderate Major Depression with Anxiety Symptoms: A Randomized, Double-Blind, Double-Dummy, Controlled, Multicenter, Parallel-Treatment Trial," *Journal of Traditional Chinese Medicine*, 39(3), 410-417. PMID: 32186013.

Zhang, Y., Han, M., Liu, Z., Wang, J., He, Q., and Liu, J. (2012, August). "Chinese Herbal Formula Xiao Yao San for Treatment of Depression: A Systematic Review of Randomized Controlled Trials," *Evidence-Based Complementary and Alternative Medicine*, 931636. doi: 10.1155/2012/931636.

Zhao, S., Hu, S., Sun, K., Luo, L., and Zeng, L. (2023, March 6). "Long-Term Pu-erh Tea Consumption Improves Blue Light-Induced Depression-Like Behaviors," *Food & Function*, 14(5), 2313-2325. doi: 10.1039/d2fo02780a.

Selhub, E.M., Logan, A.C., and Bested, A.C. (2014, January 15). "Fermented Foods, Microbiota, and Mental Health: Ancient Practice Meets Nutritional Psychiatry," *Journal of Physiological Anthropology*, 33(1), 2. doi: 10.1186/1880-6805-33-2.

Dong, X., Yang, C., Cao, S., et al. (2015). "Tea Consumption and the Risk of Depression: A Meta-Analysis of Observational Studies," *Australian & New Zealand Journal of Psychiatry*, 49(4), 334-345. doi: 10.1177/0004867414567759.

Rothenberg, D.O., and Zhang, L. (2019, June 17). "Mechanisms Underlying the Anti-Depressive Effects of Regular Tea Consumption." *Nutrients*, 11(6), 1361. doi: 10.3390/nu11061361.

Jin, Z., and Juan, Y.-K. (2021, May). "Is Fengshui a Science or Superstition? A New Approach Combining the Physiological and Psychological Measurement of Indoor Environments," *Building and Environment*, 201, 9-10. doi: 10.1016/j.buildenv.2021.107992.

Gao, S., and Handley-Schachler, M. (2003). "The Influences of Confucianism, Feng Shui and Buddhism in Chinese Accounting History," *Accounting History Review*, 13, (1), 41-68.

Kryžanowski, Špela. (2021, May 25). "Impact of Feng Shui Bedrooms on Self-Assessed Sleep and Well-Being: A Randomized Double-Blind Field Research with Instrumental Biocommunication." *South East European Journal of Architecture and Design*, 1-8. doi: 10.3889/SEEJAD.2021.10057.

Xu, Kai. *Shuowen Jiezi Xizhuan*. Beijing: Zhonghua shuju, 1987. p. 306.

Chapter 6

Scheid, V. (2013, March). "Depression, Constraint, and the Liver: (Dis)assembling the Treatment of Emotion-Related Disorders in Chinese medicine." *Cult Med Psychiatry*, 37(1), 30-58. doi: 10.1007/s11013-012-9290-y.

Su, R., Fan, J., Li, T., Cao, X., Zhou, J., Han, Z., and Ma, Y. (2019, June). "Jiawei Xiaoyao Capsule Treatment for Mild to Moderate Major Depression with Anxiety Symptoms: A Randomized, Double-Blind, Double-Dummy, Controlled, Multicenter, Parallel-Treatment Trial," *Journal of Traditional Chinese Medicine*, 39(3), 410-417. PMID: 32186013.

Klevebrant, L., and Frick, A. (2022, January-February). "Effects of Caffeine on Anxiety and Panic Attacks in Patients with Panic Disorder: A Systematic Review and Meta-Analysis," *General Hospital Psychiatry*, 74, 22-31. doi: 10.1016/j.genhosppsych.2021.11.005.

Nobre, A.C., Rao, A., and Owen, G.N. (2008). "L-theanine, a Natural Constituent in tea, and Its Effect on Mental State," *Asia Pacific Journal of Clinical Nutrition*, 17 Suppl 1, 167-8. PMID: 18296328.

Weerawatanakorn, M., He, S., Chang, C.H., Koh, Y.C., Yang, M.J., and Pan, M.H. (2023, September 5). "High Gamma-Aminobutyric Acid (GABA) Oolong Tea Alleviates High-Fat Diet-Induced Metabolic Disorders in Mice," *ACS Omega*, 8(37), 33997-34007. doi: 10.1021/acsomega.3c04874.

Hepsomali, P., Groeger, J.A., Nishihira, J., and Scholey, A. (2020, September 17). "Effects of Oral Gamma-Aminobutyric Acid (GABA) Administration on Stress and Sleep in Humans: A Systematic Review," *Frontiers in Neuroscience*, 14, 923. doi: 10.3389/fnins.2020.00923.

Hinton, T., Jelinek, H.F., Viengkhou, V., Johnston, G.A., and Matthews, S. (2019, March 26). "Effect of GABA-Fortified Oolong Tea on Reducing Stress in a University Student Cohort," *Frontiers in Nutrition*, 6, 27. doi: 10.3389/fnut.2019.00027.

Huai, J., Hui, X., Yan, D., Xu, W., Lin, D., Xiong, J., Jiang, Q., and Zhang, M. (2020, January). "Five-Element Music Relieves the Anxiety and Insomnia of Medical Staff Against COVID-19 in the Period of Medical Observation in a Single Recuperation Center in China," *QAI Journal for Healthcare Quality and Patient Safety*, 2(1), 15-18. doi: 10.4103/QAIJ.QAIJ_1_21

Chapter 7

Daumann, J., Koester, P., Becker, B., Wagner, D., Imperati, D., Gouzoulis-Mayfrank, E., and Tittgemeyer, M. (2011, January 15). "Medial Prefrontal Gray Matter Volume Reductions in Users of Amphetamine-Type Stimulants Revealed by Combined Tract-Based Spatial Statistics and Voxel-Based Morphometry," *NeuroImage*, 54(2), 794-801.

Chapter 8

Wong, A.C., et al. (2023, October 26). "Serotonin Reduction in Post-Acute Sequelae of Viral Infection," *Cell*, 186(22), 4851-4867.e20. doi: 10.1016/j.cell.2023.09.013.

Qi, D., Wong, N.M.L., Shao, R., Man, I.S.C., Wong, C.H.Y., Yuen, L.P., Chan, C.C.H., and Lee, T.M.C. (2021, July). "Qigong Exercise Enhances Cognitive Functions in the Elderly via an Interleukin-6-Hippocampus Pathway: A randomized active-controlled trial," *Brain, Behavior, and Immunity*, 95, 381-390. doi: 10.1016/j.bbi.2021.04.011.

Kim, M., Mok, H., Yeo, W.S., Ahn, J.H., and Choi, Y.K. (2021, September). "Role of Ginseng in the Neurovascular Unit of Neuroinflammatory Diseases Focused on the Blood-Brain Barrier," *Journal of Ginseng Research*, 45(5), 599-609.

Chen, Z., Zhang, Z., Liu, J., Qi, H., Li, J., Chen, J., Huang, Q., Liu, Q., Mi, J., and Li, X. (2022, April 25). "Gut Microbiota: Therapeutic Targets of Ginseng Against Multiple Disorders and Ginsenoside Transformation," *Frontiers in Cellular and Infection Microbiology*, 12:853981. doi: 10.3389/fcimb.2022.853981.

Dimpfel, W., Mariage, P.A., and Panossian, A.G. (2021, February 25). "Effects of Red and White Ginseng Preparations on Electrical Activity of the Brain in Elderly Subjects: A Randomized, Double-Blind, Placebo-Controlled, Three-Armed Cross-Over Study." *Pharmaceuticals (Basel)*, 14(3), 182. doi: 10.3390/ph14030182.

Park, K.C., Jin, H., Zheng, R., Kim, S., Lee, S.E., Kim, B.H., and Yim, SV. (2019, September). "Cognition enhancing effect of panax ginseng in Korean volunteers with mild cognitive impairment: a randomized, double-blind, placebo-controlled clinical trial," *Translational and Clinical Pharmacology*, 27(3), 92-97. doi: 10.12793/tcp.2019.27.3.92.

Scholey, A., Ossoukhova, A., Owen, L., Ibarra, A., Pipingas, A., He, K., Roller, M., and Stough, C. (2010, October). "Effects of American Ginseng (Panax quinquefolius) on Neurocognitive Function: An Acute, Randomised, Double-Blind, Placebo-Controlled, Crossover Study," *Psychopharmacology (Berl)*, 212(3), 345-56. doi: 10.1007/s00213-010-1964-y.

About the Author

NINA CHENG is the founder of The Eastern Philosophy, a traditional Chinese medicine online apothecary, with one of the largest accounts on social media in Asian medicine, accumulating over 150 million video views. She also serves as an officer of The International Association for the Study of Traditional Asian Medicine (IASTAM), the foremost community of scholars and practitioners devoted to understanding the history and contemporary practice of Asian medicines, and publisher of the journal *Asian Medicine*. She is currently studying history of medicine at the Johns Hopkins Graduate School of Medicine. Her mission is to introduce Chinese medicine to the West, substantiated with high-quality evidence- and source-based research, while staying authentic to the culture of the practice.

About the Contributors

Brandt Stickley

Brandt Stickley is a doctor of Chinese medicine with twenty-five years of clinical experience and is considered an authority on the synthesis of psychology and classical Chinese medicine. A graduate of Cornell University and American College of Traditional Chinese Medicine, he is an associate professor of classical Chinese medicine at National University of Natural Medicine (NUNM) and serves as a visiting professor at Pacific Rim College, Academy of Chinese Culture and Health Sciences, Dragon Rises College of Oriental Medicine, Yo San University, and Five Branches University, where he is creator and lead professor of the Chinese Medicine Psychiatry and Trauma-Informed Practice certificate program. He studied with his late mentor, Dr. Leon Hammer, MD, who helped develop the Shen-Hammer method of pulse diagnosis, for over twenty years.

Alexus McLeod

Alexus McLeod is a professor of philosophy at Indiana University, with a focus on areas including early Chinese philosophy and philosophical issues in the history of medicine. He has published nine books, including *The Dao of Madness* (Oxford University Press, 2021), which explores the concept of *kuang* (madness) in Confucian, Daoist, syncretist, and medical texts in early China, and its development from early moralizing discussions to its medicalization in the early Han Dynasty. Dr. McLeod received his PhD from the University of Connecticut. He served as president of the International Society for Comparative Studies of Chinese and Western Philosophy and is the editor of the journal *The Philosophical Forum*.

Shanshan Gao

Shanshan Gao is a historian and practitioner of Chinese medicine. She received her PhD at City University of Hong Kong and her bachelor of medicine as well as master of clinical medicine degrees from Beijing University of Chinese Medicine. Her research interests include the intergenerational transmission of knowledge and ideas as well as the intellectual exchange between East Asia and the Euro-American world. Dr. Gao completed her PhD dissertation titled "Forging Basic Theories for Chinese Medicine in the Early People's Republic of China: An Examination of Jingluo and Wuxing" and is currently working on article projects related to her PhD research, as well as her first book.

Daniel Spigelman

Daniel Spigelman began his Chinese medicine studies in Sydney, Australia, completed his studies at the Beijing University of Chinese Medicine, and is an inner door disciple of the Zhang Ce lineage of Wu Xing Tong Bei style of martial arts from Sun Xiangyong in Beijing. He worked in private clinical practice as well as at the National Institute of Complementary Medicine and at the Kinghorn Cancer Centre as part of a multidisciplinary oncology team. In 2017, he co-founded the Purple Cloud Institute and hosts the *Purple Cloud Podcast*, where he interviews Chinese medicine practitioners and historians.

Index